A HANDBOOK OF CHILDHOOD ANXIETY MANAGEMENT

With warm affection and esteem,
this book is dedicated by the editors to
Dr Surinder Mohan Marwah,
formerly Head of the Department of Social
and Preventative Medicine
and Dean of the Faculty of Medical Sciences,
the Institute of Medical Sciences,
Banaras Hindu University, Varanasi, India
and subsequently retired Professor, Community Medicine,
King Faisal University, Saudi Arabia.

A Handbook of Childhood Anxiety Management

Edited by
Kedar Nath Dwivedi
Ved Prakash Varma

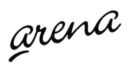

Published by
Arena
Ashgate Publishing Limited
Gower House
Croft Road
Aldershot
Hants GU11 3HR
England

Ashgate Publishing Company
Old Post Road
Brookfield
Vermont 05036
USA

British Library Cataloguing in Publication Data

A handbook of childhood anxiety management
　1. Anxiety in children
　I. Dwivedi, Kedar Nath II. Varma, Ved P. (Ved Prakash),
　1931–
　618.9'28'5223

Library of Congress Catalog Card Number: 96-86162

ISBN 1 85742 304 6

Printed and bound in Great Britain by
Hartnolls Limited, Bodmin, Cornwall

Contents

About the authors

Dino Cirelli, CQSW, BEd, is currently a member of Northamptonshire Education Department's School Phobia Assessment and Intervention Service, having held this post since its beginning in 1992. Formerly working for the Northamptonshire Education Welfare Service, over the last 13 years he has been involved very closely with pupils, families and schools in the area of school attendance. During the last six years, he has also worked as a sessional student counsellor for Leicester University's Counselling Service.

Alec Clark is UKCP-registered. He qualified as a psychiatric social worker in 1970, and worked in mainstream social services and then adult psychiatry until 1978, when he became a Sheldon Fellow in the Family Therapy Programme at the Tavistock Clinic. From 1980 to 1989, he was Principal Social Worker and Family Therapist at Kettering Child and Family Guidance Clinic. In 1989, he became a freelance therapist and trainer, specialising in the aftermath of childhood abusive experiences.

Dr Catherine Coffey graduated from Trinity College, Dublin, and later embarked on a career in psychiatry in Cork. Following general psychiatric training in Nottingham, she pursued specialist training in child psychiatry in Leicester, where she currently works as Consultant Child Psychiatrist at the Child and Family Psychiatric Service, Westcotes House.

Dr Kedar Nath Dwivedi, MBBS, MD, DPM, FRCPsych, is Consultant in Child, Adolescent and Family Psychiatry at the Child and Family Consultation Service and the Ken Stewart Family Centre, Northampton and is also Clinical Teacher in the Faculty of Medicine, University of Leicester. He graduated in medicine from the Institute of Medical Sciences, Varanasi, India, and served as Assistant Professor in Preventive and Social

Medicine in Simla before coming to the UK in 1974. Since then, he has worked in psychiatry, and is a member of more than a dozen professional associations, including the Transcultural Psychiatry Society and the Group Analytic Society, and has contributed extensively to the literature (nearly forty publications), including editing the well-received book, *Group Work with Children and Adolescents* (1993, Jessica Kingsley) and co-editing *Meeting the Needs of Ethnic Minority Children* (1995, Jessica Kingsley) and *Depression in Children and Adolescents* (in press, Whurr). He teaches on the Midland Course on Groupwork and Family Therapy and is the Director of Courses on Groupwork with Children and Adolescents in Northampton. He is also interested in Eastern, particularly Buddhist, approaches to mental health.

Dr Mary Ellis was Child and Adolescent Psychiatrist at Milton Keynes for ten years. She is now retired and working part-time, with a special interest in using a cognitive and behavioural approach in treating children and adolescents.

Mrs Mary Gray, NNEB, is currently working as Play Therapist for the Council on Addiction in Northampton, and has a very long experience of working with children in education, social services and health environments. She has studied play therapy at Roehampton and Hull, and in her work, she offers individualised programmes incorporating focused play, drama, art and music.

Dr Susanna Isaacs Elmhirst, MBBS, MD, MRCP, FRCP, FRCPsych, is a Member of the Institute of Psycho-analysis and has been the Vice-President of the British Psycho-analytic Society (1981–86). She has worked in several capacities, including being Associate Professor of Clinical Child Psychiatry at the University of Southern California (1974–80), and Consultant Child Psychiatrist at the Child Guidance Training Centre, London (1981–86). Since 1994, she has been Chair of the Ethical Committee of the British Psycho-analytic Society.

Dr Anthony C. James, MBBS, MRCP, MRCPsych, MPhil, is Consultant Psychiatrist at the Highfield Family and Adolescent Unit of the Warneford Hospital, Oxford, and Clinical Lecturer at the University of Oxford. He has a special interest in psychotic disorders and eating disorders in adolescents, and has contributed to the literature on a variety of topics, including hyperactivity, suicide and deliberate self-harm, and borderline personality disorder in adolescence.

Dr David Jones, BSc, PhD, CPsychol, is Senior Lecturer in Psychology at Birkbeck College, University of London. He is also a clinical psychologist and a family therapist. He is an Honorary Member of the Institute of Family Therapy, and is Course Director for the joint IFT/Birkbeck College MSc in Family Therapy. He has a long-standing interest in psychometrics.

Dr Raj H. Kathane, MBBS, DPM, Dip Psychother, MRCPsych, is a Consultant in Child, Adolescent and Family Psychiatry in Bedford. He has lectured at local and national conferences to different professional audiences on varied subjects, and he also teaches family therapy. His interest in hypnotherapy goes back several years, and he has received formal training in this area. A family man, his interests include classical music, photography, walking and work for charity.

Sally Letts, BSc (Hons), is currently Education Support Worker with the School Phobia Assessment and Intervention Service, part of the Northamptonshire Support Teaching and Educational Psychology Service, having held this post since its inception in 1992. She was formerly in charge of an education department hostel, a residential unit for boys with emotional difficulties and problems in attending school. She has served with the county council since 1984, with extensive experience of working with children, their families and school systems.

Dr Vaman G. Lokare, BA, MA, MPhil, PhD, ABPsS, is an Emeritus Director of Clinical Psychology in Surrey. He graduated from the University of Bombay, joined the NHS Clinical Psychology Department at the University of Southampton, and then moved to West Park Hospital, Epsom, as the Head and then the Director of the Clinical Psychology Department. He has published numerous articles in professional journals, contributed to professional books and presented several research papers at international conferences. He has been a Member of the New York Academy of Sciences and has recently guest-edited a special cross-cultural issue of *Counselling Psychology Quarterly*. Currently, he is involved with transcultural studies, and takes an active part in the work of charities.

Dr Chinta Mani, MBBS, MRCPsych, has been Consultant Psychiatrist in Learning Disabilities at Kirklands Hospital, Bothwell, Scotland, since 1987. He graduated in medicine from Panjabi University, Patiala, India, and after serving in the Panjab Health Service for four years, came to the United Kingdom in 1987. He has worked in psychiatry since 1979, and his present job involves dealing with psychiatric problems of people of all ages with learning disabilities.

Dr Jason Maratos is a Consultant Psychiatrist working with the Department of Child and Adolescent Mental Health in High Wycombe. He practises group psychotherapy and group analysis within the NHS and privately. He is a Training Group Analyst with the Institute of Group Analysis, London. He has written and lectured in the UK and abroad on matters which are of special interest to him, such as self-psychology, attachment theory, organisational dynamics and transcultural issues.

Dr Renuka Nagraj works as Consultant Child and Adolescent Psychiatrist at the Child and Family Psychiatric Service in Aylesbury, Buckinghamshire. She did her basic medical training in Madras, India. Her further training in psychiatry, and later in child psychiatry, was based in the Oxford region. Her main areas of interest are in working with bereaved children and their families, and with children who have chronic or life-threatening illnesses.

Dr Anthony Roberts is Consultant in Child and Adolescent Psychiatry at Kettering, Northamptonshire. He has a particular interest in the practice of cognitive therapy and family therapy. He is currently exploring the use of information technology as an aid both to the sharing of information and also to the facilitating of communication between healthcare professionals on a worldwide basis. His e-mail address is 100424.2525 @compuserve.com.

Dr Ved Prakash Varma, PhD, was formerly an educational psychologist with the Institute of Education, University of London, the Tavistock Clinic, and the London Boroughs of Richmond and Brent. He has edited or co-edited more than thirty books on education, psychology, psychiatry, psychotherapy and social work, and he is an international figure in the area of special needs.

Foreword

The 'age of anxiety' has proved to be a well-deserved epithet for the psychological and social insecurities of adult life in the 20th century. Sadly, as we approach the millenium, this phrase becomes more and more applicable to the world of childhood and adolescence.

Gone, it would seem, for many of today's children, is that golden age of psychologically carefree and innocent pleasures we associate with growing up. And here we are talking about anxiety as a state of mind, a deep-seated consciousness of psychological insecurity. Of course, we only have to read Dickens to appreciate how many children from another age had their childhood hijacked by grim exploitation and deprivation. But there seems to be a different quality and an insidious pervasiveness about the insecurity of life for our children in the 1990s. The source of much of it for young people in their impressionable years stems from their parents' concerns and worries. Many children experience an emotional 'hothouse', brought about by the break-up of their homes, often following long and bitter conflict between parents they love. Divorce rates are soaring. Another form of 'hothousing' is the inexorable pressure on children to achieve academically, an understandable, if undesirable, survival strategy by parents who perceive the diminishing job opportunities available to their offspring.

What bears down most heavily on children in contemporary society is a sense of living in an unsafe world, one in which violence, bullying (and worse) at school and outside it is commonplace, and one in which adults are not people to turn to as providers of protection when parents are not available, but a species to avoid as potential sources of harm. As we see it today, it is the child with psychological deficits who approaches strangers in a friendly manner. Abuse of various kinds undoubtedly existed in previous eras, but the consciousness of its existence and prevalence is drummed into the minds of children – not surprisingly when in 1994 there were 34,900 names of children under 18 years of age on the Child Protection Register in England. What else but anxiety (for sensitive, imaginative children) can be their responses to the images of hatred and hostility they are bombarded with daily on television?

The figures speak for themselves. As we see in Chapter 1 of this book, anxiety disorders are among the most prevalent forms of psychopathology during childhood and adolescence. Their consequences are serious in the short and long term; their causes are complex.

Fortunately, we have, in the *Handbook of Childhood Anxiety Management*, an invaluable guide to the vast literature (theoretical and practical) on the nature of childhood anxiety, its causes and cures. The editors have assembled an impressive team of experts to introduce practitioners and students in the various helping professions to a readable account of the complexities of this important subject.

Martin Herbert
Professor of Clinical and Community Psychology
University of Exeter

Preface

In discussing with and learning from a large number of colleagues from a variety of professional backgrounds working with children and adolescents, I have been acutely aware of the scarcity of quality practical material to help professionals help children and adolescents with their problems of anxiety today. Therefore, when Dr Varma invited me to be the first editor of this book, there could be only one response: yes! Having already edited or co-edited 30 well-received books, including *Anxiety in Children* (1984, Methuen), he brought with him an invaluable wealth of experience, wisdom and expertise to the small editorial team.

As all the contributions to the book have been of such a high quality, it has been an immense pleasure to help create this important book in meeting a long-felt need. Also, to work so collaboratively with such a diverse multidisciplinary team of experts has been particularly challenging, exciting, rewarding and educational. This team has included specialists in child, adolescent and family psychiatry, the psychiatry of learning disabilities, psychologists, and workers from school phobia assessment and intervention services.

Both Dr Varma and myself are deeply indebted to all the contributors, some of whom had to put up with our 'gentle' reminders or requests for revisions. We are equally grateful to Jo Gooderham and the team at Arena for their enthusiastic, sensitive, creative and painstakingly thorough approach to this very important project.

I am also grateful to my colleagues at the Child and Family Consultation Service and the Ken Stewart Family Centre, Child Health Directorate, Northampton General Hospital NHS Trust, for their encouragement and support. I am particularly thankful to Naina Sadrani, who has also been the dynamic centre of the service. My special thanks to Carol Weller from our library, and also to Dorothy Stephen, the Librarian, and Nicola

Buckby in the library, as their team has been most helpful in coping with so many of my 'a.s.a.p.' requests.

The essential support and the emotional nourishment from my family has also been an important ingredient for me in this project. In fact, this book marks a very auspicious time in our family: the wedding (in Varanasi, India) of our elder son, Amitabh, a hard-working junior doctor in Bristol, to Amrita, who is studying monoclonal antibodies for her PhD in London. In parallel with the creation of this book, I have also been helping organise the arrangements for the wedding through 'remote control', many thousands of miles away. As we tried to make it as traditionally Indian as possible (for example, arranging for an auspicious Indian elephant to grace the occasion), the task became more and more complex, yet equally exciting, memorable and fruitful!

Finally, we would all like to thank the reader for taking the trouble to read this book.

Kedar Nath Dwivedi

Professor Marwah's inspiring contributions

It is a real pleasure to write an appreciation of Professor Marwah, who has been an international figure in the field of health service delivery, health promotion and maternal and child health (including child mental health). I am delighted that the editors are dedicating this invaluable book in his honour.

In India some four decades ago, a new era in public health education was ushered in with the recommendations of the Medical Council of India. The then Departments of Public Health and Hygiene were converted to the Departments of Social and Preventative Medicine (SPM). Chairs of SPM were created to replace the part-time teachers of public health and hygiene. Although broad guidelines of the new curriculum for teaching the subject were provided by the Medical Council, the details and its translation into practice were left to the newly-created departments. While most medical schools still continued to teach old concepts with a few modifications, some of them took the initiative of bringing about the required reforms in public health teaching and training in medical schools. One of the few schools which took up the challenge and initiated curriculum development in response to the changed needs was the Institute of Medical Sciences, Banaras Hindu University, Varanasi. The Department of SPM at Banaras Hindu University advocated and evolved, through experimentation, community-based, integrated teaching of the subject. The curriculum developed was not only innovative but conceptually sound. This received wide approval among the SPM faculty, and was quickly adopted by other medical schools in the country, with minor adaptations to suit the local requirements.

The architect of this new curriculum was Professor Surinder Mohan Marwah, who was the first Professor and the Head of the Department of SPM at Banaras Hindu University, Varanasi, a position he held until he voluntarily relinquished the post in January 1981 to take up an assignment as Professor of Community Medicine, Faculty of Medical Sciences, King Faisal University, Saudi Arabia. What was really remarkable was the fact that Professor Marwah developed community-based, integrated teaching in SPM when hardly any such model existed anywhere. His deep conviction in the philosophy of community as a ward and the family as a bed for the teaching of SPM was the guiding principle in the evolution of this model.

Professor Marwah knew that the new discipline would achieve recognition and status among the faculty of older disciplines in the medical schools only if it was backed by research and documentation. He initiated a large number of community-based studies enquiring into the health status of rural, urban and university communities and the variables which influence them. The spectrum of his research was wide, covering subjects like the epidemiology of communicable diseases, family health, maternal and child health, family planning, nutrition and environmental health. A prolific writer, he was able to chronicle his experiences and research findings, contributing over a hundred scientific research papers and publishing several monographs.

One of the most innovative research operations which he formulated and launched was the delivery of primary healthcare. In 1979, in collaboration with the International Planned Parenthood Federation/Family Planning Association of India, he launched a project for community-based distribution of contraceptives. Covering a population of about 1.2 million in about 1,100 villages in one of the least developed areas in India, the study aimed to demonstrate that unmet family planning and primary healthcare needs can be met by utilising the community's own resources. This was a unique experiment in community participation in the delivery of primary healthcare and family planning together.

Professor Marwah believed that SPM was a multifaceted discipline and needed input from non-medical disciplines as well. Through his advocacy and strong arguments, he prevailed upon the university to create faculty posts in biostatistics, sociology and health education within the Department of SPM. This helped to set norms for other medical schools in the country.

Under his dynamic leadership, the Department of SPM made all-round progress and was recognised as one of the best in the country. In the mid-1970s, when Indo-British university collaboration was proposed for development of teaching and research activities in community medicine, the University Grants Commission selected the department at Varanasi for collaboration from the Indian side.

Professor Marwah founded the *Indian Journal of Preventive and Social Medicine* in the late 1960s. This fulfilled the academic needs of scientists at a time when there was no journal on the subject in which they could publish their research findings. He was the editor of the journal during the first ten years, and ensured that it attained a high academic standing among the scientific community. His multifaceted contributions to the subject were instrumental to a very large extent in the discipline of SPM gaining acceptance and recognition from the medical fraternity in the country. His deep sense of conviction and commitment to the discipline is still a source of inspiration to his colleagues and students.

For his contributions to the discipline of social and preventive medicine, Professor Marwah was honoured by being awarded Fellowships of the Faculty of Community Medicine of the Royal College of Physicians (UK), the National Academy of Medical Sciences (India), the Indian Public Health Association, and many other academic institutions. He has been the recipient of several orations, including the prestigious B.C. Das Gupta Oration of the Indian Public Health Association. But the best tributes paid to him, in my judgement, have been from his students, in whom he has instilled a sense of scientific enquiry, conviction and dedicated efforts in pursuing community health goals, such as the dedication of this important book, *A Handbook of Childhood Anxiety Management.*

Dr Ishwar Chandra Tiwari,
Professor of Social and Preventative Medicine, Varanasi,
Professor of Community Medicine, Joss, Nigeria (1982–84),
Adviser to the Planning Commission, Government of India (1991–93),
and Consultant, UNICEF, New Delhi, India

1 Introduction

Kedar Nath Dwivedi

It seems that anxiety is a part of the very essence of the human condition. Ibor (1969) highlights on the one hand that repetition, an aspect of anxiety, is anchored to biology and is related to the tendency to regress, and that this tendency exists in all manifestations of primeval life; on the other hand, he wonders why today we feel more condemned to anxiety than before.

Alan Watts (1983) in his book, *The Wisdom of Insecurity: A Message for an Age of Anxiety*, looks at Western society today:

> There is, then, the feeling that we live in a time of unusual insecurity. In the past hundred years or so many long-established traditions have broken down – traditions of family and social life, of government, of the economic order, and of religious belief. As the years go by, there seem to be fewer and fewer rocks to which we can hold, fewer things which we can regard as absolutely right and true, and fixed for all time. (p.14)

> Consequently our age is one of frustration, anxiety, agitation, and addiction to 'dope'. Somehow we must grab what we can while we can, and drown out the realization that the whole thing is futile and meaningless. This 'dope' we call our high standard of living, a violent and complex stimulation of the senses, which makes them progressively less sensitive and thus in need of yet more violent stimulation. We crave distraction – a panorama of sights, sounds, thrills, and titillations into which as much as possible must be crowded in the shortest possible time. (p.20)

In this volume, we are mainly concerned with pathological anxiety. Ibor (1969) distinguishes between the normal and pathological:

> The schema customarily used postulates that, although anxiety belongs to the dynamics of everyday life, there are specific conflicting situations where

1

anxiety breaks out like an eruption ... If one troubles the other disturbs. (p.163)

There has been a steady advancement over the last decade in the recognition, understanding and management of anxiety disorders throughout the lifespan. During childhood and adolescence, anxiety disorders are among the most prevalent forms of psychopathology, with prevalence rates estimated between 7.5% and 21% (Anderson et al., 1987; Bell-Dollan & Brazeal, 1993; Bernstein & Borchardt, 1991; Kashani & Orvaschel, 1988; Klein, 1994). Orvaschel and Weissman (1986), in their review of the epidemiological studies of anxiety in children, found that anxiety symptoms are, on the whole, more prevalent in girls than boys, although there is considerable variation as a function of the age of the child and the type of anxiety.

Anxiety disorders may interfere with sustained attention in the classroom, acceptance of authority, and social participation with classmates and teachers. Difficulties with concentration can disrupt the learning of new and complex academic tasks, and social withdrawal can obstruct normal interactions with peers. Thus the anxiety symptoms can have long-term detrimental effects on cognitive and social development, and are often associated with a variety of school, family and other social problems, with low self-esteem, depression, somatic distress, substance abuse, and so on (Kashani & Orvaschel, 1990).

Ialongo et al. (1995) have demonstrated that it is possible to make a reliable and valid assessment of anxiety in children as young as 5 or 6 years old, and have disputed the notion that anxiety symptoms in young children are merely transient developmental phenomena; their longitudinal study shows clear and enduring relationships with later adaptive functioning, and highlights the need to develop adequate child mental health services for their treatment and prevention.

There is also an intricate relationship between depression and anxiety disorders. In fact, in about two-thirds of children with depressive disorders, there is a history of anxiety disorders preceding depression. Similarly, there are sufficient anxiety symptoms to meet the criteria of anxiety disorder in some 40% of children with depressive disorders (Kovacs et al., 1989). This may reflect the fact that anxiety predisposes to depression, and/or anxiety and depression may reflect different evolutionary periods of the same disorder (Goodyer et al., 1991).

There appears to be a strong link between separation anxiety in childhood and adjustment problems in adulthood, a lifetime vulnerability for multiple anxiety disorders and also for certain specific anxiety disorders in adult life, especially panic disorder and agoraphobia (Lipsitz et al., 1994). It now seems to be established that the childhood onset of anxiety syndromes foreshadows adult anxiety disorders. This has also led to the refinements of classification in DSM-IV (American Psychiatric Association, 1994) in such a way that childhood and adult disorders are more closely aligned.

Looking at the contributory factors in the genesis of anxiety disorders in children and adolescents, one finds a very complex interplay of biological and environmental forces converging. The understanding of these disorders has progressed enormously in recent years through the application of human genetic research methods, especially family genetic studies and twin studies. The evidence so far indicates an interaction between genetic liability and environmental factors in the ontogeny of anxiety disorders (Alsobrook & Pauls, 1994). Childhood anxiety appears to aggregate in families, but its transmission can be explained both in terms of genetic as well as environmental effects. Thapar and McGuffin (1995) estimated the heritability rate to be 59% in an additive genetic model in their study of twins using parent-rated anxiety symptoms. In the same study, familial transmission could also be accounted for by shared environmental factors alone, when self-rated anxiety symptoms in adolescents were analysed.

The tendency to withdraw from novelty or to approach it appears to be an enduring temperamental trait (Biederman et al., 1995). The influences on the relationship between neurocognitive functioning and anxiety work both ways. Thus impaired neurocognitive functions increase anxiety, and anxiety disorders influence neurocognitive functions. The neuro-developmental aspects also play an important role in the evolution of anxiety disorders. Investigations on both animals and human beings emphasise the central role of the limbic system structures, especially the amygdala and hippocampus and connecting structures, in the modulation of anxiety (Gray, 1982; Trimble, 1988). The hippocampal formation plays an important role not only in anxiety but also in memory and new learning (Hooper & March, 1995).

Shaffer et al. (1985) have demonstrated a relationship between anxiety symptoms and neurological findings, particularly 'soft' signs. (Certain neurological signs that tend to run a developmental course and do not have a clear locus of origin are often known as soft signs: for example, general clumsiness, mirror movements, involuntary movements of choreic or athetoid type, difficulty in performing rapid alternating movements, and so on.) Similarly, a relationship between medical illnesses (and hospitalisations) and anxiety disorders has also been suggested (Lansky et al., 1975; Sermet, 1974).

Orbach et al. (1992), in their study of the emotional impact of frightening stories on children, emphasise the fact that anxiety is elicited even by the frightening elements of a story. Thus exposure to stressful life events, and to fiction, may contribute to anxiety or its disorders in a vulnerable child. Children of anxious mothers have been identified to be at a high risk of anxiety disorders, especially in the presence of inhibited temperament and attachment difficulties (Manassis et al., 1995). Early experiences of separation from parents and the influence of parental personality, overprotectiveness and transmission of anxiety from parents have therefore been suggested to play a major role. Emotionally traumatic experiences and major disruptions in children's pattern of attachment are the most common causes of anxiety disorders. For example, in a study by Gittelman-Klein and Klein (1980), severe separation anxiety was shown to have occurred following the illness or death of a loved one, a move of the child's home or a change of school in 80% of the children and adolescents.

Not only family life but also school life can be full of stressors: competition, bullies, making presentations, homework, parental pressure to achieve, fear of failure, worries about taking tests or performing in front of a large audience, and so on. When children's performance does not live up to the parent or teacher's expectation, the children are likely to suffer from high levels of evaluation anxiety. Similarly, for many children, test anxieties can be very distressing.

In addition, peer relationships have a reciprocal link with anxiety. Goodyer et al. (1989) have shown that anxious and depressive disorders are significantly more common in those school-age children who report moderate-to-poor friendships in their own lives.

There are now a number of instruments available to measure the nature and severity of the stressors and anxiety in a child's life. For example, in Axis IV of the DSM-III-R classification system (American Psychiatric Association, 1987), a scale is provided to quantitatively measure the severity of the psychosocial stressors for children and adolescents. It is a six-point scale, ranging from 'none' (i.e. no acute events or enduring circumstances that may be relevant to the disorder) to 'catastrophic' (e.g. physical or sexual abuse, chronic life-threatening illness, death of one or both parents). Similarly, there are two Coddington Life Events Scales (Coddington, 1983), one for children (aged 6–11 years) and the other for adolescents (aged 12 years and over). The focus is mainly on acute events, but the various events are assigned relative weights derived empirically from relative severity estimates by professionals. Assessment of stress from the child's perspective can be carried out using the Feel Bad Scale (Lewis et al., 1984). There are also scales to measure more specialised stressors, such as the Test Anxiety Scale for Children (Spielberger et al., 1978).

Knowledge and experience in managing anxiety disorders in children and adolescents have also advanced substantially in recent years. There are a variety of approaches that have constantly been refined. Many of these – namely cognitive behavioural therapy, play therapy, psychodynamic psychotherapy, family therapy, hypnotherapy, group therapy and pharmacotherapy – are presented in this volume. Their usage (either singly or in some combination) depends upon the needs of the particular child and the resources and the skills available in the service. It really is amazing how much relief can be achieved by simple but skilled treatment.

When Nathan, a 10-year-old boy, was referred to our service, he had a variety of anxiety-related, severely handicapping symptoms. He had an intense fear of germs, which led to rituals of excessive washing, avoidance of touching a whole range of objects (such as shoes, door knobs, stair gates) and refusal to eat due to fear of vomiting. Paul Sellwood, the therapist, gradually managed to engage him in therapy (the nature of this problem can also obstruct therapy). The turning point came when Nathan managed to draw a huge picture of a germ, and then, with the encouragement of the therapist, turned it into a 'very silly germ'. From then onwards, various exposure exercises, including 'playing in mud in the back garden' and so on, became gradually and miraculously possible.

The problem now is not so much the lack of a body of therapeutic knowledge but the resources for their implementation. There is an urgent need to evolve comprehensive services so that there is early and appropriate intervention (Dwivedi, 1993). Early intervention would not only improve adjustment during childhood but would also reduce the incidence of emotional distress and disability during adulthood. Several recent surveys of the child mental health services have highlighted the enormous gaps (Kurtz, 1992; Kurtz et al., 1994). Parry-Jones (1992) underlines:

> evidence of prolonged lack of funding, resulting in marked shortfall of manpower by any standards and in poor working conditions, rendering child and adolescent psychiatry a truly 'Cinderella' service. Under such circumstances, opportunities for involvement in less urgent clinical activities, such as preventive or health promotion programmes, are likely to be absent or minimal. (p.5)

There is now at least a recognition of the urgent need to build up an appropriate infrastructure for child mental health services at different levels (primary, secondary and tertiary), offering a comprehensive (promotive, preventive, curative and rehabilitative) service in a collaborative fashion (between various departments such as health, social services, education, the Home Office), as highlighted in recent official documents (NHS Health Advisory Service, 1995; Audit Commission, 1994).

References

Alsobrook, J.P. & Pauls, D.L. (1994) 'Genetics of anxiety disorders', *Current Opinion in Psychiatry,* 7(2), pp.137–9.

American Psychiatric Association (1987) *Diagnostic and Statistical Manual of Mental Disorders: Third Edition-Revised (DSM-III-R),* Washington, DC: American Psychiatric Association.

American Psychiatric Association (1994) *Diagnostic and Statistical Manual of Mental Disorders: Fourth Edition (DSM-IV),* Washington, DC: American Psychiatric Association.

Anderson, J.C., Williams, S., McGee, R. & Silva, P.A. (1987) 'DSM-III disorders in preadolescent children: Prevalence in a large sample from the general population', *Archives of General Psychiatry,* 44(1), pp.69–76.

Audit Commission (1994) *Seen But Not Heard,* London: HMSO.

Bell-Dollan, D. & Brazeal, T.J. (1993) 'Separation anxiety disorder, overanxious disorder, and school refusal', *Child and Adolescent Psychiatric Clinics of North America,* 2, pp.563–80.

Bernstein, G.A. & Borchardt, C.M. (1991) 'Anxiety disorders of childhood and adolescence: A critical review', *Journal of the American Academy of Child and Adolescent Psychiatry,* 30(4), pp.519–32.

Biederman, J., Rosenbaum, J.F., Chaloff, J. & Kagan, J. (1995) 'Behavioural inhibition as a risk factor for anxiety disorders', in March, J.S. (ed.) *Anxiety Disorders in Children and Adolescents,* New York: Guilford Press.

Coddington, R.D. (1983) 'Measuring the stressfulness of a child's environment', in Humphrey, J.H. (ed.) *Stress in Childhood,* New York: AMS Press, pp.97–126.

Dwivedi, K.N. (1993) 'Group work in child mental health services', in Dwivedi, K.N. (ed.) *Group Work with Children and Adolescents,* London: Jessica Kingsley, pp.290–306.

Gittelman-Klein, R. & Klein, D.F. (1980) 'Separation anxiety in school refusal and its treatment with drugs', in Hersov, L. & Berg, I. (eds) *Out of School,* London: John Wiley, pp.321–41.

Goodyer, I., Wright, C. & Altham, P. (1989) 'Recent friendships in anxious and depressed school age children', *Psychological Medicine,* 19(1), pp.165–74.

Goodyer, I., Germany, E., Gowrusankur, J. & Altham, P. (1991) 'Social influences on the course of anxious and depressive disorders in school-age children', *British Journal of Psychiatry,* 158, pp.676–84.

Gray, J.A. (1982) *The Neuropsychology of Anxiety: An Inquiry into the Functions of the Septo-hippocampal System,* Oxford: Oxford University Press.

Hooper, S.R. & March, J.S. (1995) 'Neuropsychology', in March, J.S. (ed.) *Anxiety Disorders in Children and Adolescents,* New York: Guilford Press.

Ialongo, N., Edelsohn, G., Werthamer-Larsson, L., Crockett, L. & Kellam, S. (1995) 'The significance of self-reported anxious symptoms in first grade children: Prediction to anxious symptoms and adaptive functioning in fifth grade', *Journal of Child Psychology and Psychiatry,* 36(3), pp.427–37.

Ibor, J.J.L. (1969) 'Anxiety and its importance in psychiatry', in Lader, M.H. (ed.) *Studies of Anxiety,* Ashford, Kent: Headley Brothers, pp.163–6.

Kashani, J.H. & Orvaschel, H. (1988) 'Anxiety disorders in mid-adolescence: A community sample', *American Journal of Psychiatry,* 145(8), pp.960–4.

Kashani, J.H. & Orvaschel, H. (1990) 'A community study of anxiety in children and adolescents', *American Journal of Psychiatry,* 147(3), pp.313–18.

Klein, R.G. (1994) 'Anxiety disorders', in Rutter, M., Taylor, E. & Hersov, L. (eds) *Child and Adolescent Psychiatry: Modern Approaches* (3rd edn), Oxford: Blackwell Scientific Publications, pp.351–74.

Kovacs, M., Gatsonis, C., Paulauskas, S.L. & Richards, C. (1989) 'Depressive disorders in childhood, IV: A longitudinal study of comorbidity with and risk for anxiety disorders', *Archives of General Psychiatry,* 46(9), pp.776–82.

Kurtz, Z. (ed.) (1992) *With Health in Mind: Mental Health Care for Children and Young People,* London: Action for Sick Children.

Kurtz, Z., Thomes, R. & Wolkind, S. (1994) *Services for the Mental Health of Children and Young People in England: A National Review. Report to the Department of Health,* London: South West Thames Regional Health Authority.

Lansky, S.B., Lowman, J.T., Voto, T. & Gyulay, J. (1975) 'School phobia in children with malignant neoplasms', *American Journal of the Disabled Child,* 129, pp.42–6.

Lewis, L.E., Siegel, J.M. & Lewis, M.A. (1984) 'Feeling bad: Exploring sources of distress among preadolescent children', *American Journal of Public Health,* 74(2), pp.117–22.

Lipsitz, J.D., Martin, L.Y., Mannuzza, S., Chapman, T.F., Liebowitz, M.R., Klein, D.F. & Fyer, A.J. (1994) 'Childhood separation anxiety disorder in patients with adult anxiety disorders', *American Journal of Psychiatry,* 151(6), pp.927–9.

Manassis, K., Bradley, S., Goldberg, S., Hood, J. & Swinson, R.P. (1995) 'Behavioural inhibition, attachment and anxiety in children of mothers with anxiety disorders', *Canadian Journal of Psychiatry,* 40(2), pp.87–92.

NHS Health Advisory Service (1995) *Together We Stand: Child and Adolescent Mental Health,* London: HMSO, Department of Health, Science and Education.

Orbach, I., Vinkler, E. & Har-Even, D. (1992) 'The emotional impact of frightening stories on children', *Journal of Child Psychology and Psychiatry,* 33(3), pp.379–89.

Orvaschel, H. & Weissman, M.M. (1986) 'Epidemiology of anxiety disorders in children: A review', in Gittelman, R. (ed.) *Anxiety Disorders of Childhood,* London: Guilford Press, pp.3–72.

Parry-Jones, W. (1992) 'Management in the National Health Service in relation to children and their provision of child psychiatric services', *ACPP Newsletter,* 14(1), pp.3–10.

Sermet, O. (1974) 'Emotional and medical factors in child mental anxiety', *Journal of Child Psychology and Psychiatry,* 15(4), pp.313–21.

Shaffer, D., Schonfeld, I., O'Connor, P.A., Stokman, C., Trautman, P., Shafer, S. & Ng, S. (1985) 'Neurological soft signs: Their relationship to psychiatric disorder and intelligence in childhood and adolescence', *Archives of General Psychiatry,* 42(4), pp.342–51.

Spielberger, C.D., Gonzalez, H.P., Taylor, C.J., Algaze, B. & Anton, W.D. (1978) *Examination Stress and Test Anxiety,* Washington, DC: Hemisphere.

Thapar, A. & McGuffin, P. (1995) 'Are anxiety symptoms in childhood heritable?', *Journal of Child Psychology and Psychiatry,* 36(3), pp.439–47.

Trimble, M. (1988) 'The neurology of anxiety', *Postgraduate Medical Journal,* 64(Supplement 2), pp.22–6.

Watts, A. (1983) *The Wisdom of Insecurity: A Message for an Age of Anxiety,* London: Rider.

2 Epidemiology of anxiety disorders

Catherine Coffey

Introduction

There can be little doubt that child psychiatry, as Graae (1990) has expressed it, 'relative to adult psychiatry ... is in an earlier stage of describing itself'. Much of the information already to hand with regard to emotional and psychological disturbances in children results from the application of adult-derived data to concepts and situations that apply to children, because of an apparent overlap between these populations in at least some of their experiences. However, over the past two decades, growing doubt has been increasingly supported by evidence which suggests a lack of equivalence between the experiences of children and adults, and the need for wider exploration of how developmental stage interacts with the expression of psychopathology and the subjective and objective experiences of it.

The ubiquitous experience of anxiety leads to a sense of familiarity with the topic, and indeed, anxiety-related disorders are the most frequent cause for children and adolescents consulting a child psychiatric service. However, the precise continuity or relationship between the 'normal' fears of childhood and pathology, either during the same period or subsequently in adulthood, remains as yet to be elucidated. Bell-Dolan et al. (1990), in their review of anxiety symptoms in normal children, refer to the findings of Lapouse and Monk in their paper of 1959, in which they report the finding that 43% of mothers of 6–12-year-old children described their children as having seven or more fears or worries; 41% felt that these fears or worries were recurring.

Marks, in his review of developmental fears (Marks, 1987), observed that normal children 'have fears that rise and fall in a predictable sequence at particular phases of development'. He attributed these fears

9

to the result of the interaction between genes and environment, and believed that some fears were innate, arising without prior experience of the situation, others arising in the presence of some tiny trigger (prepotent, i.e. dormant until a certain trigger exerts its effect). Examples cited included fears of heights, strangeness and separation, reflecting their particular evolutionary relevance. Fears progress from those of strangers and separation from 6 months of age, through fears of animals at 2–4 years, to fears of darkness, imaginary creatures and storms from 4 to 6 years. Fear of strangers and strange peers persisting beyond 29 months were described by Marks as potentially persisting into adulthood as shyness.

A few fears, such as those of sex, agoraphobia and failure, were referred to as arising principally in adolescence. Marks described fear of blood-injury and animals as fears which, when found in adults, had usually persisted from childhood; those animal phobias which arose in adult life he regarded as rare, and usually the result of a trauma such as a dog bite. Longitudinal prospective studies of general child populations will be essential in order to determine the nature of any continuity that may exist between these developmental sequences and the experience and expression of pathology.

Communication remains the key issue for all aspects of emotional disorders, whether between patient and physician in determining the relief offered, or between professionals attempting to elaborate a formal and consistent means by which knowledge may be defined and shared. Thus since the 1950s, we have become increasingly familiar with the efforts of the American Psychiatric Association and the World Health Organisation, in the forms of the *Diagnostic and Statistical Manual*, DSM-II, III, III-R and IV, and the *International Classification of Diseases*, ICD 8, 9 and 10. That there are two such major classificatory systems is testimony to the complexity of the task, as well as the relative inadequacy of available definitive research data to act as guidance. Epidemiological data clearly require agreement between professionals as to how conditions will be defined and thus diagnosed.

Attempts at classification initially related principally to those disorders described in adult patients. With regard to anxiety disorders, the inclusion in DSM-II of disorders of childhood and adolescence led to increased attention being focused on the definition of disorders across this developmental period. Observations from studies such as that of Lapouse and Monk (1959), which led to their conclusion that the symptoms of children were 'transient and innocuous', have been supplanted by comprehensive evaluation of those fears and worries which are within the developmental repertoire of most children, and the attributes which lead clinicians to more confidently assert the presence of pathology. Community studies have been vital in procuring such data, but in their turn have raised doubts as to the certainty with which we feel we can generalise about disorders between clinic populations, and those disorders coincidentally uncovered in community samples.

Both the ICD and DSM classificatory systems offered categorical means by which adult psychopathology might be defined. In 1968, it was suggested that certain disorders existed which appeared to have their principal expression in childhood, and accordingly, these were included within both systems. Within DSM-III, reference was made to disorders first evident in infancy, childhood or adolescence. These included the following anxiety disorders:

- separation anxiety disorder (SAD);
- avoidant disorder of childhood or adolescence (AD);
- overanxious disorder (OAD).

With subsequent revisions of the DSM systems, the value of separate classification has been closely scrutinised, and in conjunction with focused research studies, the most recent version, DSM-IV, refers only to separation anxiety disorder in this distinct group. Overanxious disorder and avoidant disorder have been included within generalised anxiety disorder and social phobia respectively. The 'adult' section of anxiety disorders includes criteria for generalised anxiety disorder (GAD), social phobia, specific (simple) phobia, panic disorder (PD), agoraphobia, obsessive-compulsive disorder (OCD), post-traumatic stress disorder (PTSD) and anxiety disorder not otherwise specified. The required criteria are applied to children and adolescents with some modifications with regard to duration of symptoms, as well as the number of essential criteria demanded for diagnosis.

The dilemma as to whether or not it is appropriate to apply adult diagnostic criteria in attempting such diagnoses in children and adolescents continues. Central to this question is the role of cognitive development in the presentation of any anxiety disorder, and thus the range of symptoms that can reasonably be demanded in determining caseness. The danger of relying totally on the account of responsible and familiar adults has frequently been described, with the expected lowered prevalence figures for 'internalising disorders', such as anxiety, than if the child's account were also to be included. A good understanding of cognitive development is thus a prerequisite in attempting to anticipate the impact this might have on any proposed system of classification, when applied to children and adolescents.

Instruments

In his review of the classification of childhood disorders, Werry (1991) draws attention to the need for more definite and coherent knowledge with which to guide disposal of ever-diminishing resources for child psychiatric patients. Risk and protective factors, treatment outcomes and suitable populations for these treatments, along with clearer under-standing of the long-term consequences of disorders, are essential com-ponents of this knowledge base. Developing taxonomic systems which offer reliability, internal consistency, specificity, external validity as well as utility, in conjunction with appropriate methods of data capture, are fundamental to this task. Werry comments that there is now available a 'solid set of epidemiological studies relating to the prevalence of child psychiatric disorder'.

Categorical systems such as DSM and ICD have afforded opportunities to clinicians to incorporate intuitive, clinically-derived hypotheses into systems which can now be subjected to empirical testing. In conjunction with dimensional systems which use empirical, multivariate statistical approaches to group symptoms, opportunity is now afforded for the provision of data which more closely reflect the information gathered routinely by the clinician and utilised in the formulations of diagnoses, treatment and outcome measures. There has been a significant improve-ment in the availability of interviews and assessment schedules with established psychometric validity and reliability for use in child and adolescent populations.

Hodges (1993), in her comprehensive review of the use of six structured interviews with children, concluded that:

1 Children and adolescents can respond to questions which enquire about their mental status.
2 There was no indication of morbidity or mortality risks associated with such enquiries.
3 Parent and child reports are not interchangeable.
4 Self-report questionnaires are insufficient for (a) subject selection and (b) outcome measurement when the presence or absence of clinical symptomatology is of interest.

With regard to the third point, Hodges refers to the work of Achenbach et al. (1987), who observed that agreement between informant accounts depended on the type of pathology under scrutiny: behavioural symp-toms generated more agreement, depressive symptoms elicited only moderate concordance, and there was poor agreement for anxiety symp-toms. Silverman and Eisen (1992) and Last and Hersen (1987) described better agreement for anxiety symptoms if the population was originally referred for treatment of an anxiety disorder. Hodges concludes, therefore, that in researching child and adolescent disorders, both child and adult reports are needed. Bernstein and Borchardt (1991) also draw attention to the impact of age and developmental level on the nature of the data collected by child interview, given the apparent increased frequency of certain anxiety disorders at different ages.

In her review, Hodges outlines the current status of interview schedules and their various origins, referring principally to the CAPA (Child and Adolescent Psychiatric Assessment), CAS (Child Assessment Schedule), DICA (Diagnostic Interview for Children and Adolescents), DISC (Diagnostic Interview Schedule for Children, plus its revisions, DICA-R and DICA 2), ISC (Interview Schedule for Children) and the KSADS (Schedule for Affective Disorders and Schizophrenia for School Aged Children). Four of these interviews were developed at about the same time: the ISC and KSADS arose out of research on depression, and the CAS and DICA were developed for use with paediatric and psychiatric samples. The DISC was specifically developed for epidemiological research. The most recently introduced interview, the CAPA, has as yet little established psychometric data available. Both the ISC and KSADS generate diagnoses in a clinically-derived manner. This entails the use of information from the child as well as the adults involved, and thus requires decisions with regard to the weights given to the different information sources, as well as to whether or not the child merits a diagnosis of disorder. The other interviews referred to above provide a level of objectivity, in that diagnoses can be generated via computer algorithms. Thus diagnosis can be decided by computer and based on child or adult data only, or on a combination of the two.

The psychometric data available for these interviews for anxiety disorders suggest that poorer-reliability data exist for the diagnosis of these disorders compared to the diagnosis of depression or attention deficit disorder, and the least reliable for the DISC. Validity measures similarly reflect weak data, especially for anxiety disorders. Hodges remarks on the relative lack of data with regard to symptom scales, which might potentially be sources of continuous variables which indicate the extent of symptoms. She also emphasises that the use of these interviews is extremely labour-intensive, thus making the essential large-scale population studies employing these instruments expensive and time-consuming.

Despite the economical ease of administration of such self-report measures as the Children's Depression Inventory (CDI), State-Trait Anxiety Inventory for Children (STAIC) and Youth Self-report (YSR), significant limitations mean that generally, interview schedules are primarily

Table 2.1   DSM-III diagnoses

Study	Instrument	Prevalence of disorder
Anderson et al. (1987) New Zealand birth cohort	DISC-C Rutter A & B	17.6% 11-year-olds 12% – SAD, OAD, S + Soc P, Depn & Dysthy
Links et al. (1989) Ontario Child Health Survey	SDI CBCL	11% 4–11 years 14% 12–16 years G 5% 12–16 years B
Bell-Dolan et al. (1990) 'Normal' children	KSADS, CDI FSSC-R, RCMAS, STAIC, LS	41% 6–12 years worry of separation 43% mothers of 6–12 years report 7+ fears/child
Kashani and Orvaschel (1990) School population	CAS, RCMAS CAS-P	4.8% Anx: C+P 13.8% Anx: CAS-P 21% Anx: CAS
Whitaker et al. (1990) Epidemiological study	Part I: ESI, EAT, BDI LOI-C Part 2: DICA, ISC	0.6% – PD 1.9% – OCD 3.7% – GAD 4.0% – MDD 4.9% – Dysthy
McGee et al. (1990) Population study	DISC–C	22% >/= 1 disorder 5.9% – OAD
McGee et al. (1992) Longitudinal community study	DISC-C, Rutter A & B at 11 years DISC-C + RPBC at 15 years	42% at 11 years any disorder, also had disorder at 15 years × 2 increased prev anxiety disorder from 11 to 15 years

Key to abbreviations

Instruments

BDI	Beck Depression Inventory
CAS	Child Assessment Schedule
CAS-P	Child Assessment Schedule – Parent Version
CBCL	Child Behaviour Checklist
CDI	Children's Depression Inventory

Key to abbreviations *continued*

DICA	Diagnostic Interview for Children and Adolescents
DISC	Diagnostic Interview Schedule for Children
EAT	Eating Attitude Test
ESI	Eating Symptoms Inventory
FSSC-R	Fear Survey Schedule for Children – Revised
ISC	Interview Schedule for Children
KSADS	Schedule for Affective Disorders and Schizophrenia for School Aged Children
LOI-C	Leyton Obsessional Inventory – Child Version
LS	Loneliness Scale
RCMAS	Revised Children's Manifest Anxiety Scale
RPBC	Revised Problem Behaviour Checklist
Rutter A	Rutter Child Scale A
Rutter B	Rutter Child Scale B
STAIC	State-Trait Anxiety Inventory for Children
SDI	Survey Diagnostic Instrument

Disorders

Depn	Depression
Dysthy	Dysthymia
GAD	Generalised Anxiety Disorder
MDD	Major Depressive Disorder
OAD	Overanxious Disorder
OCD	Obsessive-Compulsive Disorder
PD	Panic Disorder
S	Simple Phobia
SAD	Separation Anxiety Disorder
Soc P	Social Phobia

used. Diagnoses, primary and comorbid, are reliably made, the importance of which for treatment outcome has been alluded to by Pliszka (1992). Stavrakaki et al. (1987a) remark on the benefits of including rating scales such as the Achenbach Child Behaviour Checklist (CBCL), Revised Children's Manifest Anxiety Scale (RCMAS) and Brief Psychiatric Rating Scale (BPRS) when conducting studies, from their experience of examining concordance between informants with regard to anxiety and depressive disorders in children. Reliability and validity data have been well established for the use of the RCMAS scale with children and adolescents in the work of Reynolds and Richmond (1978).

Loeber et al. (1989) suggest the use of parent or adult as informant for those externalising disorders such as attention deficit disorder and oppositional disorder. Children, in their view, could be regarded as better informants for internalising disorders, for example separation anxiety disorder, overanxious disorder and dysthymic disorders. The study of

Verhulst and Van der Ende (1992) of 883 adolescents from the general population also suggested the superiority of the adolescents' own account of internal thoughts and feelings compared with that from their parents. Silverman and Eisen (1992) caution that developmental stage must also be considered when assessing anxiety disorders. In their study of 50 out-patients and their parents, they found that 6–9-year-olds were unreliable reporters of anxiety symptoms, but were reliable with regard to simple fears. With increasing age, they noted that reliability of children's anxiety accounts increased. The results of application of some of the available interviews in a number of studies are summarised in Table 2.1.

Fears

Ollendick et al. have published widely on the prevalence of fears in the general population of children and adolescents in Britain and in a number of other countries. Using a modification of the survey devised by Scherer and Nakamura (1968), Ollendick et al. utilised the Fear Survey Schedule for Children with children from areas as geographically diverse as the USA, Australia, Britain and Hong Kong (Ollendick et al., 1985, 1989, 1991; Dong et al., 1995). They consistently observed an age-related decline in reported fears, as well as a gender difference in the numbers of fears reported at a particular age, in that girls repeatedly indicated more fears than boys. King et al. (1989) argue from their study of fears in 8–16-year-old children that this apparent sex difference in reporting of fears may reflect the response of children to gender-role expectations rather than revealing genuine differences in fear responsiveness, and refer to the work of Graziano et al. (1979) to support their view.

In the studies of Ollendick et al., the 'top ten' fears generally relate to situations of danger and life-threatening circumstances. Minimal differ-ences were recorded between children in Australia and the USA, and similarly between youngsters in Britain. For British children, the tenth fear of USA peers came eleventh in their league: fear of illness. Earth-quakes was an additional fear included for UK subjects. McGee et al. confirmed these findings in their 1990 study of a birth cohort in New Zealand, from whom they recorded fears at 11 and 15 years of age. Their results demonstrated a fall in the number of reported fears up to age 11, but showed a subsequent rise, possibly post- or peri-pubertally. Younger children referred to fears of the dark, heights and animals, while older children recorded fears relating to 'social and agoraphobic' situations.

The continuity from childhood fears to disorders, and in particular anxiety disorders later in childhood or adulthood, awaits further clarifica-tion. Ollendick et al. (1991), in their study of British children, observed that highly-fearful children possessed lower self-concepts and were more external in their locus of control. They employed the Children's Depression Inventory, Revised Children's Manifest Anxiety Scale and the FSSC-R referred to earlier to record children's fears, as well as to estimate the presence of anxiety and/or depressive disorder. A moderate relationship between fears recorded and presence of anxiety was observed, with only a modest relationship between fears and depression. They queried the uniqueness of constructs to fears, anxiety and depression. This point bears special relevance to the issue of comorbidity discussed later.

Anxiety

Much if not all of the research data currently available utilises those categories of anxiety disorder described in DSM-III and DSM-III-R referred to earlier. Thus overanxious disorder, avoidant disorder of childhood or adolescence and the third and only one of the three retained in DSM-IV, separation anxiety disorder, receive considerable attention, with regard to their prevalence as well as the validity of regarding these childhood disorders as distinct from similar disorders in adults. A variety of study approaches has been used in the research cited below, and the diversity of methodology employed, as well as that within the population types examined, demands considerable caution in the interpretation of the data recorded and the inferences drawn.

Bernstein and Borchardt (1991) summarise much of the data now available with reference to:

- prevalence figures;
- demographic profiles;
- comparison of clinical presentation for differing age groups;
- patterns of comorbidity.

They consider differences between clinic and non-clinic populations, and the dangers of extrapolating between these potentially very dissimilar groups. They regard the use of validated, structured interviews as improving homogeneity within populations identified with disorders. They also refer to the impact of informant source on the nature and attributable value of information so obtained. Costello (1989a), Kashani and Orvaschel (1990) and McGee et al. (1990), in their different studies, found variations in prevalence rates depending on the specific informant, child or adult. They also observed that prevalence rates increased as the number of informants used to make a judgement of diagnosis rose.

That some anxiety disorders are found in particular age groups is illustrated by their inclusion of the findings of Geller et al. (1985) and Ryan et al. (1987), who noted a higher prevalence for separation anxiety disorder in prepubertal as compared with postpubertal children.

In their review, Bernstein and Borchardt (1991) also emphasise the use in some studies of impairment criteria, essential for some DSM-IV and DSM-III-R diagnoses, but also consider this issue from the perspective of not converting symptom presence into 'disorder'.

With regard to prevalence rates of specific disorders, they refer to the large-scale study of Anderson et al. (1987), who conducted a longitudinal study using a birth cohort of New Zealand children, and employed the Diagnostic Interview Schedule for Children along with Rutter A and B profiles, with which DSM-III diagnoses were derived. However, no impairment, severity or duration data were recorded for diagnoses referred to as 'anxiety' and 'phobias'. Nearly 800 children were screened: 3.5% were recorded as SAD, 2.9% as OAD, 2.4% as having simple phobias and 1% as social-phobic. Of those with anxiety disorders, only 20% sought help, which compared with 8% without disorders who sought assistance.

In a follow-up of this study in 1990, McGee et al. reported a prevalence rate of almost 6% for overanxious disorder among 11-year-olds. This represented nearly half of the children with a diagnosis of anxiety. When these children were examined in turn, 50% were found to have a concurrent diagnosis of depressive or other anxiety disorder. The second most common disorder in this group was non-aggressive conduct disorder, recorded for a further 5.9%. Simple phobia was the third most commonly described disorder, at 3.6%, with the most common fears expressed being phobias related to speaking in front of the class, heights, aeroplanes and being in the water.

A Puerto Rican community survey by Bird et al. (1988) found that nearly 7% could be recorded as SAD, which reduced to a prevalence of closer to 5% when impairment criteria were required. When criteria for maladjustment were employed, their findings of 3.9% for simple phobia reduced similarly to 2.6%. Bowen et al., in their 1990 study of over 3,000 children in the Ontario Child Health Study, reported a prevalence of 3.6% for OAD and 2.4% for SAD. In a self-report study of 1,676 schoolchildren, conducted by Beitchman et al. (1989), greater frequencies for conduct-related problems were observed among boys using the Children's Self-report Questionnaire. Girls, on the other hand, scored more highly on worry, sensitivity and emotional parameters.

Bell-Dolan et al. (1990), utilising a small sample of 'never psychiatrically ill' children, attempted to elucidate further the nature of anxiety symptoms experienced by 'normal' children. They subjected 62 such children to semi-structured interview (KSADS), as well as a battery of questionnaires (FSSC-R, RCMAS), along with interviews of a parent and first-degree relative. Thus they attempted to make diagnoses in accordance with DSM recommendations, in both subjects and relatives. They wished to explore whether the anxiety experiences of normal children were qualitatively different from those of children with disorders, or whether their symptoms differed only in quantity and severity. With regard to the presence of fears in children, they demonstrated the age-related decline observed by Ollendick et al. (1989). Younger children responded to those sudden, intense and novel stimuli, fears of separation and the supernatural. Older children were more preoccupied by fears of school, and peer- and health-related situations. Girls reported more fears than boys, and these included fears of illness, animals and injury, while boys described fears of academic and economic failure. Girls were also more likely to experience more than one anxiety disorder. Older children recorded overanxious disorder more frequently, while younger children experienced separation anxiety disorder.

Bell-Dolan et al. (1990) drew particular attention to a subgroup of children referred to by them as the 'sub-clinically anxious group'. These children had symptoms of anxiety which did not merit the diagnosis of a disorder, but appeared to have distinctive attributes, particularly with regard to the apparent prevalence of psychopathology in first-degree relatives. Sixty-nine per cent of their fathers were reported as depressed and suffering from alcohol abuse. The authors raise the possibility of this group retaining an increased risk of developing disorder later in childhood or adulthood, as well as the dilemma of the nature–nurture continuum. While elaborating many intricate and pertinent questions and possible answers from their data, Bell-Dolan et al. (1990) acknowledge the disproportionate number of data analyses conducted, compared with their sample sizes. They observe that self-report questionnaires, unstructured clinical interviews and structured diagnostic interviews all identify somewhat different groups of children. They also question whether current diagnostic methods miss anxiety disorders in children when they exist, particularly where children may be considered by experienced clinicians as anxious, but themselves isolate affect to the extent that they fail to report the experience of anxiety.

Kashani and Orvaschel (1990) reported on their cross-sectional study of 210 8-, 12- and 17-year-old school-goers. Using the CAS and the RCMAS, they found a prevalence of 21% for anxiety disorder, using child-generated data, nearly 14% with parent-derived data, and nearly 5% when both child and parent scores were combined. OAD increased in prevalence across the age range, with 8-year-olds registering a prevalence of 8.6%, 11.4% for the 12-year-old group, and 17% for the 17-year-old group. Over 36% of this sample who were identified as having anxiety disorder were found to have two or more diagnosable anxiety disorders, using the CAS.

Velez et al. (1989) interviewed almost 800 children and their parents, and found that this yielded a prevalence of 5.4% for SAD and 2.7% for OAD. A similar study by Costello et al. (1989a) yielded 4.1% and 4.6% respectively for the same categories, despite the younger lower age of inclusion of 7–11 years.

Whitaker et al. (1990) conducted a two-stage epidemiological study of over 5,000 children, with one of the specific objectives being to provide a sufficiently large sample size for the less common disorders such as obsessive-compulsive disorder. Utilising a self-report screening test, they identified 470 children for further interview. They describe their results for panic disorder, 0.6% (over 5 per thousand), and a prevalence of almost 2% for OCD. Figures for GAD were recorded as 3.7%, with that for dysthymia approaching 5%. Children in this sample were aged between 13 and 18 years.

Panic

In their review of panic disorder in children and adolescents, Ollendick et al. (1994) suggest that in order to further this study, we must accept the advice of Alessi et al. (1987), who observe that we might more usefully consider how panic disorder might be manifested in children, rather than persisting with the use of adult-derived criteria and seeking their expression in child and adolescent populations. There has been considerable debate as to the validity of the diagnosis for use with a child and adolescent population. Nelles and Barlow (1988) questioned whether, in fact, 'children experience these physiological sensations, and have the cognitive ability to misinterpret experiences and attribute them to internal causes'. They addressed this query particularly in the context of discrimination being made between those panic attacks that arise 'spontaneously' and those regarded as 'cued'. They doubt whether a child can make the necessary cognitive attribution of somatic symptoms and sensations being internally-based, and thus giving rise to spontaneous panic attacks. There is no longer a requirement for the individual to describe fears of madness or death in order for the diagnosis of panic to be made within the DSM classificatory system.

It seems that many researchers and clinicians have been comfortable to include adolescents among the ranks of potential sufferers of panic symptoms. The place of children in this group has been suggested from adult studies of panic and the somewhat unreliable retrospective accounts of onset in childhood of panic disorder or attacks.

Nelles and Barlow (1988) have compared the symptomatology of paediatric patients with hyperventilation syndromes, where the physiological symptoms resemble those found with panic but occur most frequently in the absence of the accompanying cognitive attributions. They suggest that these disorders may be precursors of more formal panic disorder.

Normative data

A number of studies have examined the prevalence of panic symptoms in non-psychiatrically-referred populations. Variations in the employed methodology compromise the generalisability of some of the findings, but offer useful indications for the direction of future research.

In a study of nearly 390 high-school students, aged 12–19, Warren and Zgourides (1988) found a prevalence of panic disorder of 4.7%; 60% regarded themselves as having experienced at least one panic attack in the past, and this was further refined to 32% using DSM-III criteria. For the majority of students responding, the panic attacks were not identified as severe or recurrent problems, although 24% feared a recurrence. The study of Macaulay and Kleinknecht (1989) also considered the severity of panic symptoms as well as their frequency. The Panic Attack Questionnaire (PAQ) was modified in order to reflect DSM-III-R diagnoses of panic, and completed by over 600 high-school students. Overall, 63% reported experiencing a panic attack some time in the previous 12 months; 76% of participating girls reported a panic attack, whereas only 47% of the boys did so. This represented a prevalence of 7.3% in girls and 3.2% in boys. Although 5.4% rated their panic symptoms as severe, only 10% were receiving treatment. Onset of symptoms was reported by this group most frequently at 13 years of age.

Hayward et al. (1989) conducted a survey of 95 14–16-year-old students, and found a lifetime prevalence of 11.6% for panic attacks with four or more symptoms. A further 3.2% reported limited-symptom attacks. Those describing panic attacks also scored more highly for depression, parental separation, and were smokers.

In a later study, Hayward et al. (1992) employed the Structured Clinical Interview for DSM-III-R Disorders to assess over 750 schoolgirls. The pubertal status of the group was also reported using self-report Tanner Staging with the Sexual Maturity Index (SMI). A prevalence of 5.3% was recorded for one four-symptom panic attack. At each age, a higher rate of panic attacks were found in the more physically mature girls. Of the 94 girls with an SMI score of 1–2, none reported any panic attacks. This contrasted with the 100 girls with SMI scores of 5, among whom a prevalence of 8% was recorded. Thus it appears that pubertal status exerts a powerful effect on the presence of panic symptoms. King et al. (1993) used the PAQ and the RCMAS with 246 13–15-year-olds and 288 subjects aged 16–18 years. They recorded a rate for one panic attack of 42%, with 'panickers' having significantly higher scores on the RCMAS. In Anderson et al.'s (1987) large New Zealand study of 11-year-olds, there were no recorded instances of panic disorder.

Clinic populations

Studies reporting on recorded incidence of panic attacks and disorder vary greatly in the age range of subjects interviewed and included, as well as in their adherence or otherwise to DSM-III-R criteria. Alessi et al. (1987) examined 61 hospitalised adolescents in their unit with the Schedule for Affective Disorders and Schizophrenia (SADS) and found that 15% had PD. A further 24% were described as 'possible PD'. Although their criteria were less rigorous than those of DSM-III-R, this does raise the question of validity with regard to the number of symptoms required for diagnosis, and the use of apparently arbitrary cut-off points. Only large prospective studies can help elucidate the significance of more or less symptoms for panic attacks and disorder, as well as most other disorders. A later study by Alessi and Magen (1988) found a prevalence of 5% for PD in 130 consecutive admissions to a child psychiatric unit. These children were reported as prepubertal (aged between 7 and 12 years), with a mean age of onset for PA of 8 years. Vitiello et al. (1990) also reported on a prepubertal population of some 1,200 outpatients and inpatients. This represented the accumulated clinic attendance over a four-year period and yielded only six cases of PD using DSM-III-R criteria.

Last and Strauss (1989) interviewed nearly 180 children and parents in their study utilising the KSADS and SCID (Structured Clinical Interview for DSM-III-R: Non-patient Version). They included children aged between 5 and 18 years, and reported a prevalence of 10% for PD. Of these 17 cases so identified, 12 were diagnosed as PD only, while the remaining 5 were PD with agoraphobia. SAD was diagnosed in 12% of this group.

Paediatric samples yield interesting data with regard to children seen with symptoms of hyperventilation. Enzer and Walker, in their 1967 examination of hospital records, identified 44 children between 5 and 16 years of age who had been referred with symptoms of hyperventilation in the absence of relevant organic pathology. Seventy per cent of this group were female, and all reported 'attacks of breathing too fast', accompanied by dizziness, syncope and paraesthesia. On assessment, it was felt that these were anxious children who reported a number of specific fears. These findings were very similar to those of Herman et al. in their 1981 study, part of a longitudinal study of hyperventilation in children attending the Mayo Clinic. They described 34 children with symptoms of rapid breathing, accelerated heart rate, lightheadedness and paraesthesiae. Of 30 children followed up, 12 still experienced problems with hyperventilation as adults. This group were further described as reporting anxiety accompanied by a sense of impending doom. Van Winter and Stickler (1984) identified six children aged between 9 and 16 with a diagnosis of PD and who described an age of onset of 8 years. This group also came from the Mayo Clinic. Herskowitz (1986) examined a group of 9–16-year-olds referred with possible neurological symptoms, four of whom were reported as having PD in conjunction with a primary neurological diagnosis. It appears that paediatric populations may harbour significant numbers of children with symptoms consistent with that of a diagnosis of at least PA and possibly PD. The evidence as yet remains bedevilled by the lack of clarity from previous studies with regard to age and pubertal status at the time of diagnosis, as well as the inadequacy of longitudinal data which might indicate which constellation of symptoms in relation to panic disorders is of most significance. It is clear that panic attack symptoms are neither uncommon nor infrequent within the general population, and of little ultimate significance for the majority of people. It is of importance to note the observations of Alessi et al. (1987) and Last and Strauss (1989), who found that panic disorder was frequently not uncovered in general psychological evaluations of adolescents referred to clinical services.

Obsessive-compulsive disorder

Thomsen (1994), in a comprehensive review of the literature, reports the conclusions from earlier studies that obsessive-compulsive disorder in children and adolescents is a rather rare disorder. These early studies have relied principally on clinic-based samples and retrospective diagnoses from adult patients. Black (1974) and others report a prevalence for OCD of between 1% and 4% from this work. Rutter et al. (1976), in their Isle of Wight study, reported a rate of 0.3% for obsessional symptoms in 10–11-year-old children.

Thomsen refers to the prevalence rates reported for the child psychiatric populations examined by Judd (1965) and Hollingsworth et al. (1980) at between 0.2% and 1.2%. McGough et al. (1993) usefully draw attention to the 'great secretiveness' which is frequently observed in child and adolescent patients with OCD symptoms, who, in their view, are frequently extremely aware that their symptoms are abnormal. They suggest that studies may significantly underestimate and underdiagnose this condition as a result.

Bouvard and Dugas (1993) allude to another dimension which confounds assessment of treatment outcome, similarly relating to the observed secretiveness of affected patients. They refer to their observations of the increased number and frequency of symptoms reported by patients as they apparently improve on medication, and the fact that patients become more forthcoming about their symptom disclosures. Flament et al. (1988), as part of the two-stage epidemiological study by Whitaker et al., examined the results of screening surveys for OCD symptoms. In all, 93 out of a total of 356 high-school students exceeded the threshold for clinical disorder on the Leyton Obsessional Inventory – Child Version. A further 188 scored for a number of obsessional symptoms but fell below the cut-off clinical threshold, while 75 were negative for all symptoms. These researchers refer to the data available from retrospective studies of adult populations, which suggest that between a third and a half of adult patients with OCD have their onset before 15 years of age. They concluded from their findings that the prevalence of OCD in the general adult population was about 0.3%, very similar to the figure of 0.2% described by Hollingsworth et al. As with the work of Bell-Dolan et al., Flament et al. are concerned by the large group whom they describe as 'sub-clinical', and whose ultimate significance with regard to OCD awaits the elucidation of prospective studies. They were also struck by the apparently low rate of intervention in those children identified as having OCD in their group, where only a fifth received help. Unlike reports of other studies, Flament et al. found no gender difference in their incidence data, whereas a male preponderance has more frequently been described.

Thomsen (1994) observes that the prevalence of OCD appears similar across cultures, with the most frequent age of onset reported as 10 years. Toro et al. (1992) comment on the high prevalence of psychiatric morbidity in first-degree relatives of children with OCD. They allude in particular to Tourette's disorder and the finding that 32% were found to have suffered tics or Tourette's syndrome. This reflects the rates reported by Leonard et al. (1992), but is disputed by Schapiro and Schapiro (1992), who criticise the mode of diagnosis where tics are regarded as compulsions, and thus a diagnosis of Tourette's reflects the inherent expectations and definitions of measurement. The apparently higher incidence of OCD in patients who subsequently receive a diagnosis of Asperger's disorder (2 out of 60) is also commented on by Thomsen, who refers to the overall high prevalence of psychiatric disorder in this group, predominantly anxiety-related.

In his 1992 paper, Thomsen refers to the work of Zeitlin (1986), who studied the continuities and discontinuities in symptomatology in patients admitted to a psychiatric hospital, both in childhood and adulthood. He characterised OCD as a psychiatric illness with a very high consistency of symptoms from childhood into adult life. Zeitlin observed that more than 70% of patients with OCD symptoms in childhood showed them again in adult life, whereas 10% of children without these symptoms first showed them as adults. Viewed from adult life, 60% of those with OCD symptoms had similar symptoms as a child, but only 5% of those without the adults' symptoms had had childhood obsessions. It is clear that much remains to be elucidated with regard to OCDs and the common neuropsychopathological pathways that might underlie their origins (Gorman et al., 1989) and the potential implications these may hold for heritability and familial forms of the disorder.

Separation anxiety disorder

From the work of Anderson et al., it appears that SAD may be regarded as one of the most common of the childhood anxiety disorders. The mean age of presentation is about 9 years, with this disorder being significantly more frequent in younger children than adolescents (Kashani & Orvaschel, 1990). Bernstein's study, reported in 1991, found that SAD occurred most frequently in subjects diagnosed as suffering from anxiety disorders only, and anxiety disorders with depressive disorders. OAD was the second most commonly diagnosed disorder. In their review of panic disorder, Ollendick et al. (1994) referred to the frequent associated finding of SAD in subjects with PD. This has led some to hypothesise the possible link between this association and the later findings in adults of PD with agoraphobia. However, insufficient longitudinal data are available to reliably comment on whether or not SAD can be regarded as a precursor of agoraphobia in some people.

Overanxious disorder

Strauss et al. (1988b), Bowen et al. (1990) and Werry (1991) had raised concerns as to the validity of this disorder as a distinct diagnosis over a number of years, and thus the inclusion of OAD within the spectrum of symptoms represented by GAD in the current version of DSM-IV represents a timely response to their warnings. The fact that many of the symptoms of GAD are common to other DSM disorders, and in particular those physiological symptoms of which a varying number are required for different diagnoses, means that the difficulty of distinguishing between comorbidity and an actual overlap of symptomatology continues.

OAD was more frequently found in the adolescent age group, and from the work of Last et al. (1987b), appeared to have an equal sex incidence. McGee et al. (1990) and Strauss et al. (1988b) found that these older children reported more symptoms than younger children, and worry about past behaviour is a frequent dominant symptom. Controlled studies are required to elucidate the precise distinction between those children with a disorder and those with the 'normal' number of anxious symptoms.

Simple and social phobias (avoidant disorder)

Avoidant disorder is now included within the adult group of social phobias. Emphasis is placed on there being discernible difficulty with peer relationships for the child, and not just being confined to those with adults. Little research is available for consideration with regard to this diagnosis. Last and Strauss (1989) found a prevalence of 4.5% in children with SAD. A further 27.3% of those with OAD were diagnosed as also suffering from 'avoidant disorder'. Strauss and Last (1993) conducted a study of phobic disorders among children referred to their anxiety disorder clinic over a 22-month period. The prevalence of phobic disorders within this group was 59%; 30% were found to suffer from DSM-III-R social phobia, 36% had simple phobias, and a further 3% agoraphobia. Social-phobic children had higher total fears scores, a greater number of intense fears, as well as more fears of failure and criticism than non-phobic children. This group also appear to consistently report more fearfulness than children with simple phobias. Strauss and Last found an equal incidence of phobia across gender, in contrast with the results from other studies such as Anderson et al. (1987), who found that social phobia was five times more common in 11-year-old girls than their male peers, and simple phobia was almost twice as frequent. In studies of comorbidity, where depressive disorders are concurrently diagnosed with anxiety disorders, social phobia is most frequently reported. This may reflect the later age of onset of social phobia, which is most often seen in adolescence. Simple phobias are seen across the age range, with some studies reporting an elevation in incidence between the ages of 10 and 13 years.

Post-traumatic stress disorder

The criteria used for diagnosis of this disorder in children and adolescents are essentially similar to those identified as requirements when making this diagnosis in adults, with modifications appropriate to the developmental level of the child. For example, recording the intrusiveness of repetitive play of affected children is frequently interpreted as representative of re-enactment of the traumatic incident(s), replacing the flashback phenomena more typical of adult accounts. Data relating to these disorders in child and adolescent populations come principally from studies of children who have been part of a major disaster (Pynoos et al., 1987) and of children who have been physically and sexually abused. It is clear that children do indeed suffer from such post-traumatic sequelae. Pynoos et al. described how the proximity to the traumatic event increased the likelihood of severe symptomatology.

Pelcovitz et al. (1994) described a study of physically-abused adolescents, and concluded that this form of abuse was more significantly associated with other psychiatric disorders such as depression and other behavioural and social difficulties. The work of Solomon suggests that inherent predispositions may exist within individuals which increase the likelihood of their developing the disorder when confronted with major stress.

Fears

These have been alluded to in detail earlier, with particular reference to the studies of Ollendick et al. Anderson et al. reported a prevalence of 2.4% in their 1987 epidemiological study, while McGee et al. (1990) recorded a prevalence of 3.6% in adolescents.

Comorbidity

A number of studies have considered the issue of comorbid diagnoses which include concurrent anxiety disorders, as well as affective and 'externalising' disorders. Evaluation of these studies is made more difficult by the differences between populations included regarding their source, some being clinic-derived, others epidemiological samples, with a wide range in the ages of subjects included for examination.

Last et al. (1987a) referred to 73 outpatients seen at their clinic for children and adolescents with anxiety disorders. They recorded a primary diagnosis of SAD in 33% of this group; a further 15% were diagnosed as OAD, another 15% as suffering from school phobia, while 15% were rated as suffering from a major depressive episode. They comment on the similarities between these findings and those described by Barlow et al. (1986) in their study of anxious adults. Bernstein (1991) offers a useful review of previous attempts to decipher the relationship between anxiety and depressive symptomatology in children and adolescents. A consistent finding in both child and adult studies appears to be the increased severity in anxiety and depressive symptoms where there is comorbidity of anxiety and depressive disorders. Strauss et al. (1988a) report increased severity in those children with depression and anxiety disorders, as indicated by their scores on the STAIC, RCMAS and the FSSC-R.

Kovacs et al. (1989) examined the prevalence of comorbid anxiety disorders in a clinic population of children aged 8–13 years and diagnosed as depressed on the ISC. They found that 41% had a comorbid anxiety disorder, SAD being most frequently recorded. They discuss the central issue of whether anxiety and depression are distinct disorders, or whether they are more accurately regarded as occupying positions on a continuum. Bernstein (1991) considers the implications of comorbidity for treatment, and observes the need for more investigations into the demographics, family histories, clinical presentations and biological markers associated with children and adolescents having comorbid anxiety and depressive disorders.

Woolston et al. (1989) discuss the comorbidity of anxiety/affective disorders and behaviour disorders, and emphasise the importance of assessing academic achievement in children from this group. Although their study consisted of a small number of inpatients, over 50% were diagnosed as having concurrent behaviour and anxiety/affective disorders, with low achievement scores. Russo and Beidel (1994) review the literature with regard to the childhood prevalence of anxiety and concurrent externalising disorders, and comment on the lack of definitive research on the effects of comorbid externalising disorders on the assessment and treatment of childhood anxiety disorders. They observe the greater than expected co-occurrence of these disorders, as reported in a number of epidemiological studies, in particular those of Anderson et al. (1987) and McGee et al. (1990). In this latter study, the data suggest that the comorbidity rate drops as the subjects mature to adolescence. This trend was also largely supported by data from clinic-referred samples. Kashani and Orvaschel (1990) describe an increase in oppositional behaviour among adolescents diagnosed with anxiety disorder. The suggestion from some studies of a relationship between parental affective/anxiety disorders and externalising disorders in their offspring awaits further elucidation.

Heritability

Moreau and Weissman (1992) included an age- and sex-matched control group in their study of over 200 offspring of depressed parents. In the seven cases of PD identified, four of the seven also had parents with PD. SAD and major depressive disorder were the principal concurrent diagnoses. Similarly, Bradley and Hood, in their 1993 study, found that 50% of parents themselves had a diagnosis of PD. Earlier reference was made to the possibility of SAD preceding PD and agoraphobia. The lack of adequate controls and longitudinal normative data with reference to pubertal status leaves considerable scope for future studies.

With regard particularly to the issue of comorbidity, Bernstein (1991) remarks on the available evidence from family history studies which have compared child probands with a history of anxiety disorders and child probands with depressive disorders. It appears that there are no significant differences in the prevalence rates of psychiatric disorders of first-degree relatives of these children. Livingston et al. (1985) examined the family histories of those children with severe anxiety disorders and those with depression. Again, both sets of relatives were found to have similar prevalence rates for affective disorders and alcoholism. In the study by Last et al. (1987c) which examined psychiatric illness in mothers of anxious children, it was found that 83% of mothers in the clinic sample with SAD/OAD had a lifetime history of OAD. Fifty per cent of these mothers presented with their disorder at the time of their child's assessment with anxiety symptoms.

Rosenbaum et al. (1992) discuss the possibility that children at high risk for the development of anxiety disorders might be identified by the presence of a temperamental characteristic described as 'behavioural inhibition to the unfamiliar'. They conducted a study of children and parents, where parents fell into three groups: (1) behavioural inhibition plus anxiety; (2) behavioural inhibition only; (3) no behavioural inhibition or anxiety in their child. In their results, they found that parents of children with behavioural inhibition and anxiety had higher rates of two or more anxiety disorders than those parents of children with behavioural inhibition only, or neither inhibition nor anxiety. They suggest that using parental anxiety loading, those children with behavioural inhibition may be used to identify children at particularly high risk for the development of childhood anxiety disorders. Further studies are clearly essential for the clarification of the factors operating which contribute to the subsequent development of anxiety in behaviourally-inhibited children.

Summary

While there have clearly been a number of well-designed and well-conducted research studies to date in the field of anxiety disorders in childhood and adolescence, the need for further large-scale studies remains. It is apparent that these disorders have a high prevalence, with an unknown course and consequence for the sufferer in many cases. The adequacy of current taxonomic systems requires further rigorous examination, with longitudinal evaluation of the stability and outcome of these derived categories.

In order that ever-diminishing resources can be focused more appropriately on those in greatest need, a clear awareness of the real incidence and prevalence of disorders is required; the significance of the interplay between environment, heredity, temperament and past experience also demands our attention. Jablensky's (1986) three principal hurdles to psychiatric epidemiology remain:

- a common language for case definition, diagnostic criteria and data classification;
- agreement with regard to standardised, widely-acceptable assessment tools;
- a common analytic technique and uniform method of data presentation.

These afford some guiding principles with which to direct urgently-required future studies.

References

Achenbach, T., McConaughy, S. & Howell, C. (1987) 'Child and adolescent behavioural and emotional problems: Implications of cross-informant correlations for situational specificity', *Psychological Bulletin*, 101, pp.213–32.
Agras, S., Sylvester, D. & Oliveau, D. (1969) 'The epidemiology of common fears and phobias', *Comprehensive Psychiatry*, 10, p.151.

Alessi, N.E. & Magen, J. (1988) 'Panic disorder in psychiatrically hospitalised children', *American Journal of Psychiatry*, 145, pp.1,450–2.

Alessi, N.E., Robbins, D.R. & Dilsaver, S.C. (1987) 'Panic and depressive disorders among psychiatrically hospitalized adolescents', *Psychiatry Research*, 20, pp.275–83.

Anderson, D.J., Noyes, R. & Crowe, R.R. (1984) 'A comparison of panic disorder and generalised anxiety disorder', *American Journal of Psychiatry*, 141(4), pp.572–5.

Anderson, J.C., Williams, S., McGee, R. & Silva, P.A. (1987) 'DSM-III disorders in preadolescent children: Prevalence in a large sample from the general population', *Archives of General Psychiatry*, 44(1), pp.69–76.

Barlow, D.H., Dinardo, P.A., Vermilyea, B.B. & Blanchard, E.E. (1986) 'Comorbidity and depression among the anxiety disorders', *Journal of Nervous and Mental Disease*, pp.63–72.

Beck, A.T., Sokol, L., Clark, D.A., Berchick, R. & Wright, F. (1992) 'A crossover study of focused cognitive therapy for panic disorder', *American Journal of Psychiatry*, 149(6), pp.778–83.

Beidel, D. (1991) 'Social phobia and overanxious disorder in school-age children', *Journal of the American Academy of Child and Adolescent Psychiatry*, 30(4), pp.545–52.

Beidel, D.C., Turner, M.W. & Trager, K.N. (1994) 'Test anxiety and childhood anxiety disorders in African-American and white school-children', *Journal of Anxiety Disorders*, 8(2), pp.169–79.

Beitchman, J.H., Wekerle, C. & Hood, J. (1987) 'Diagnostic continuity from preschool to middle childhood', *Journal of the American Academy of Child and Adolescent Psychiatry*, 26(5), pp.694–9.

Beitchman, J.H., Kruidenier, B., Inglis, A. & Clegg, M. (1989) 'The Children's Self-Report Questionnaire: Factor score age trends and gender differences', *Journal of the American Academy of Child and Adolescent Psychiatry*, 28(5), pp.714–22.

Bell-Dolan, D.J., Last, C.G. & Strauss, C.C. (1990) 'Symptoms of anxiety disorders in normal children', *Journal of the American Academy of Child and Adolescent Psychiatry*, 29(5), pp.759–65.

Berg, I., Marks, I., McGuire, R. & Lipsedge, M. (1974) 'School phobia and agoraphobia', *Psychological Medicine*, 4, pp.428–34.

Bernstein, G.A. (1991) 'Comorbidity and severity of anxiety and depressive disorders in a clinic sample', *Journal of the American Academy of Child and Adolescent Psychiatry*, 30(1), pp.43–50.

Bernstein, G.A. & Borchardt, C.M. (1991) 'Anxiety disorders of childhood and adolescence: A critical review', *Journal of the American Academy of Child and Adolescent Psychiatry*, 30(4), pp.519–32.

Bernstein, G.A. & Garfinkel, B.D. (1986) 'School phobia: The overlap of affective and anxiety disorders', *Journal of the American Academy of Child and Adolescent Psychiatry*, 25(2), pp.235–41.

Biederman, J. (1987) 'Clonazepam in the treatment of pre-pubertal children with panic-like symptoms', *Journal of Clinical Psychiatry*, 48(Supplement), pp.38–41.

Biederman, J., Rosenbaum, J.F., Bolduc-Murphy, E.A., Faraone, S.V., Chaloff, J., Hirshfeld, D.R. & Kagan, J. (1993) 'A 3-year follow-up of children with and without behavioural inhibition', *Journal of the American Academy of Child and Adolescent Psychiatry*, 32(4), pp.814–21.

Bird, H.R., Gould, M.S. & Staghezza, B. (1992) 'Aggregating data from multiple informants in child psychiatry epidemiological research', *Journal of the American Academy of Child and Adolescent Psychiatry*, 31(1), p.78.

Bird, H.R., Canino, G., Rubio-Stipec, M. & Gould, M.S. (1988) 'Estimates of prevalence of childhood maladjustment in a community survey in Puerto Rico', *Archives of General Psychiatry,* 45, p.1,120.

Birmaher, B., Waterman, G.S., Ryan, N., Cully, M., Balach, L., Ingram, J. & Brodsky, M. (1994) 'Fluoxetine for childhood anxiety disorders', *Journal of the American Academy of Child and Adolescent Psychiatry,* 33(7), pp.993–9.

Black, A. (1974) 'The natural history of obsessional neurosis', in Beech, H.R. (ed.) *Obsessional States,* London: Methuen, pp.19–54.

Black, B. & Robbins, D.R. (1990) 'Panic disorder in children and adolescents', *Journal of the American Academy of Child and Adolescent Psychiatry,* 29(1), pp.36–44.

Bouvard, M. & Dugas, M. (1993) 'Fluoxitine in obsessive-compulsive disorder in adolescents', *International Clinical Psychopharmacology,* 8(4), pp.307–10.

Bowen, R.C., Offord, D.R. & Boyle, M.H. (1990) 'The prevalence of overanxious and separation anxiety disorder: Results from the Ontario Child Health Study', *Journal of the American Academy of Child and Adolescent Psychiatry,* 29(5), pp.753–8.

Bradley, S.J. (1990) 'Panic disorder in children and adolescents: A review with examples', *Adolescent Psychiatry,* 17, p.433.

Bradley, S.J. & Hood, J. (1993) 'Psychiatrically referred adolescents with panic attacks: Presenting symptoms, stressors, and comorbidity', *Journal of the American Academy of Child and Adolescent Psychiatry,* 32(4), pp.826–9.

Burke, J.D., Borus, J.F., Burns, B.J., Hannigan Millstein, K. & Beasley, M.C. (1982) 'Changes in children's behaviour after a natural disaster', *American Journal of Psychiatry,* 139(8), pp.1,010–14.

Costello, E.J. (1989a) 'Child psychiatric disorders and their correlates: A primary care pediatric sample', *Journal of the American Academy of Child and Adolescent Psychiatry,* 28, pp.851–8.

Costello, E.J. (1989b) 'Developments in child psychiatric epidemiology', *Journal of the American Academy of Child and Adolescent Psychiatry,* 28, p.836.

Coudert, A.J., Jalenques, I. & Geneste, J. (1991) 'Problématique parentale et anxiété de l'enfant', *Neuropsychiatrie de L'Enfance et de L'Adolescence,* 39(11–12), pp.588–91.

Cox, B.J., Endler, N.S. & Swinson, R.P. (1991) 'Panic attacks: An empirical test of a panic–anxiety continuum', *Journal of Anxiety Disorders,* 5, pp.21–34.

Dong, Q., Yong, X., Lin, L., Yang, B. & Ollendick, T.H. (1995) 'The stability and prediction of fears in Chinese children and adolescents: A one-year follow up', *Journal of Child Psychology and Psychiatry,* 36(5), pp.819–32.

Eisenberg, L. (1958) 'School phobia: A study in the communication of anxiety', *American Journal of Psychiatry,* 114, pp.712–18.

Enzer, N.B. & Walker, P.A. (1967) 'Hyperventilation syndrome in childhood', *Journal of Pediatrics,* 70(4), pp.521–32.

Ferrari, M. (1976) 'Fears and phobias in childhood: Some clinical and developmental considerations', *Child Psychiatry and Human Development,* 17(2), pp.75–87.

Flament, M.F., Whitaker, A., Rapoport, J.L., Davies, M., Berg, C.Z., Kalikow, K., Screery, W. & Schaffer, D. (1988) 'Obsessive compulsive behaviour in adolescence: An epidemiological study', *Journal of the American Academy of Child and Adolescent Psychiatry,* 27(6), pp.764–71.

Francis, G., Last, C.G. & Strauss, C.C. (1992) 'Avoidant disorder and social phobia in children and adolescents', *Journal of the American Academy of Child and Adolescent Psychiatry,* 31(6), pp.1,086–9.

Francis, G., Robbins, D.R. & Grapentine, W.I. (1992) 'Panic disorder in children and adolescents', *Rhode Island Medicine,* 75(5), p.273.

Garland, E.J. & Smith, D.H. (1991) 'Simultaneous prepubertal onset of panic disorder, night terrors, and somnambulism', *Journal of the American Academy of Child and Adolescent Psychiatry*, 30(4), pp.553–5.

Geller, B., Chestnut, E.C., Miller, M.D., Price, D.J. & Yates, E. (1985) 'Preliminary data on DSM-II associated features of major depressive disorders in children and adolescents', *American Journal of Psychiatry*, 142, pp.643–4.

Gorman, J.M., Liebowitz, M.R., Fyer, A.J. & Stein, J. (1989) 'A neuroanatomical hypothesis for panic disorder', *American Journal of Psychiatry*, 146, pp.148–61.

Graae, F. (1990) 'High anxiety in children', *Journal of Clinical Psychiatry*, 51(Supplement 18–19), p.50.

Graae, F., Milner, J., Rizotto, L. & Klein, R.G. (1994) 'Clonazepam in childhood anxiety disorders', *Journal of the American Academy of Child and Adolescent Psychiatry*, 33(3), pp.372–6.

Graziano, A.M., De Giovanni, I.S. & Garcia, K.A. (1979) 'Behavioural treatment of children's fears: A review', *Psychiatric Bulletin*, 86, pp.804–30.

Hagopian, L.P. & Slifer, K.J. (1993) 'Treatment of separation anxiety disorder with graduated exposure and reinforcement targetting school attendance: A controlled case study', *Journal of Anxiety Disorders*, 7(3), pp.271–80.

Hanna, G.L. (1995) 'Demographic and clinical features of obsessive compulsive disorder in children and adolescents', *Journal of the American Academy of Child and Adolescent Psychiatry*, 34(1), p.19.

Hayward, C., Killen, J.D. & Barr Taylor, C. (1989) 'Panic attacks in young adolescents', *American Journal of Psychiatry*, 146(8), pp.1,061–2.

Hayward, C., Killen, J.D., Hammer, L.D., Litt, I.F., Wilson, D.M., Simmonds, B. & Barr Taylor, C. (1992) 'Pubertal stage and panic attack history in fourth and fifth grade girls', *American Journal of Psychiatry*, 149, pp.1,239–43.

Herjanic, B. & Campbell, W. (1977) 'Differentiating psychiatrically disturbed children on the basis of a structural interview', *Journal of Abnormal Child Psychology*, 5, pp.127–34.

Herman, S.P., Stickler, G.B. & Lucas, A.R. (1981) 'Hyperventilation syndrome in children and adolescents: Long-term follow-up', *Pediatrics*, 67(2), pp.183–7.

Herskowitz, J. (1986) 'Neurological presentations of panic disorder in childhood and adolescence', *Developmental Medicine and Child Neurology*, pp.617–23.

Hodges, K. (1993) 'Structured interviews for assessing children', *Journal of Child Psychology and Psychiatry*, 34(1), pp.49–68.

Hollingsworth, C.E., Tangnay, P.E., Grossman, L. & Pabst, P. (1980) 'Long-term outcome of obsessive-compulsive disorder in childhood', *Journal of the American Academy of Child and Adolescent Psychiatry*, 19, pp.134–44.

Ialongo, N., Edelsohn, G., Werthamer-Larsson, L., Crockett, L. & Kellam, S. (1995) 'The significance of self-reported anxious symptoms in first grade children: Prediction to anxious symptoms and adaptive functioning in fifth grade', *Journal of Child Psychology and Psychiatry*, 36(3), pp.427–37.

Jablensky, A. (1986) 'Epidemiological surveys of mental health of geographically defined populations of Europe', in Weissman, M.M., Myers, J.R. & Ross, C.E. (eds) *Community Surveys of Psychiatric Disorders*, New Brunswick: Rutgers University Press, pp.257–313.

Jalenques, I. & Coudert, A.J. (1991) 'Reflections on the relationships between anxiety and depression in children', *Pédiatrie*, 46(11), pp.743–50.

Judd, L. (1965) 'Obsessive compulsive neurosis in children', *Archives of General Psychiatry*, 12, p.136.

Kagan, J., Reznick, J.S., Clarke, C. & Snidman, N. (1984) 'Behavioural inhibition to the unfamiliar', *Child Development*, 55, pp.2,212–25.

Kashani, J.H. & Orvaschel, H. (1990) 'A community study of anxiety in children and adolescents', *American Journal of Psychiatry,* 147(3), pp.313–18.

Kearney, C.A. & Silverman, W.K. (1992) ' "Let's not press the panic button": A critical analysis of panic and panic disorder in adolescents', *Clinical Psychology Review,* 12, p.293.

Keller, M.B., Lavori, P.W., Wunder, J., Beardslee, W.R., Schwartz, C.E. & Roth, J. (1992) 'Chronic course of anxiety disorders in children and adolescents', *Journal of the American Academy of Child and Adolescent Psychiatry,* 31(4), p.595.

King, N.J. & Tonge, B.J. (1992) 'Treatment of childhood anxiety disorders using behaviour-therapy and pharmacotherapy', *Australian and New Zealand Journal of Psychiatry,* 26(4), pp.644–51.

King, N.J., Gullone, E., Tonnge, B.J. & Ollendick, T.H. (1993) 'Self-reports of panic attacks and manifest anxiety in adolescents', *Behaviour Research and Therapy,* 31(1), pp.111–16.

King, N.J., Ollier, K., Iacuone, R., Schuster, S., Bays, K., Gullone, E. & Ollendick, T.H. (1989) 'Fears of children and adolescents: A cross-sectional Australian study using the Revised Fear Survey Schedule for Children', *Journal of Child Psychology and Psychiatry,* 30(5), pp.775–84.

Klein, D.F., Manuzza, S., Chapman, T. & Fyer, A.J. (1992) 'Child panic revisited', *Journal of the American Academy of Child and Adolescent Psychiatry,* 31(1), p.112.

Klein, R.G., Koplewicz, H.S. & Kanner, A. (1992) 'Imipramine treatment of children with separation anxiety disorder', *Journal of the American Academy of Child and Adolescent Psychiatry,* 31(1), pp.21–8.

Kovacs, M., Gatsonis, C., Paulauskas, S.L. & Richards, C. (1989) 'Depressive disorders in childhood, IV: A longitudinal study of comorbidity with and risk for anxiety disorders', *Archives of General Psychiatry,* 46(9), pp.776–82.

Kutcher, S.P., Reiter, S., Gardner, D.M. & Klein, R.G. (1992) 'The pharmacotherapy of anxiety disorders in children and adolescents', *Psychiatric Clinics of North America,* 15(1), pp.41–67.

Labatte, L.A., Pollack, M.H., Otto, M.W., Langenauer, S. & Rosenbaum, J.F. (1994) 'Sleep panic attacks: An association with childhood anxiety and adult psychopathology', *Biological Psychiatry,* 36(1), pp.57–60.

Lafreniere, P.J. & Dumas, J.E. (1992) 'A transactional analysis of early-childhood anxiety and social withdrawal', *Development and Psychopathology,* 4(3), pp.385–402.

Lapouse, R. & Monk, M. (1959) 'Fears and worries in a representative sample of children', *American Journal of Orthopsychiatry,* 29, pp.803–18.

Last, C.G. & Hersen, M. (eds) (1987) *Issues in Diagnostic Research: Developmental Considerations,* New York: Plenum Press.

Last, C.G. & Strauss, C.C. (1989) 'Panic disorder in children and adolescents', *Journal of Anxiety Disorders,* 3, pp.87–95.

Last, C.G., Strauss, C.C. & Francis, G. (1987a) 'Comorbidity among childhood anxiety disorders', *Journal of Nervous and Mental Disease,* 175(12), pp.726–30.

Last, C.G., Perrin, S., Hersen, M. & Kazdin, A.E. (1992) 'DSM-III-R anxiety disorders in children: Sociodemographic and clinical characteristics', *Journal of the American Academy of Child and Adolescent Psychiatry,* 31(6), p.1,070.

Last, C.G., Hersen, M., Kazdin, A.E., Finkelstein, R. & Strauss, C.C. (1987b) 'Comparison of DSM-III separation anxiety and overanxious disorders: Demographic characteristics and patterns of comorbidity', *Journal of the American Academy of Child and Adolescent Psychiatry,* 26(4), pp.527–31.

Last, C.G., Hersen, M., Kazdin, A.E., Francis, G. & Grubb, H.J. (1987c) 'Psychiatric illness in the mothers of anxious children', *American Journal of Psychiatry*, 144, pp.1,580–3.

Leonard, H.L., Lenane, M.C., Swedo, S.E., Rettew, D.C., Gershon, E.S. & Rapoport, J.L. (1992) 'Tics and Tourette disorder: A 2-year to 7-year follow-up of 54 obsessive-compulsive children', *American Journal of Psychiatry*, 149, p.1,244.

Links, P.S., Boyle, M.H. & Offord, D.R. (1989) 'The prevalence of emotional disorder in children', *Journal of Nervous and Mental Disease*, 177(2), pp.85–91.

Lipsitz, J.D., Martin, L.Y., Manuzza, S., Chapman, T.F., Liebowitz, M.R., Klein, D.F. & Fyer, A.J. (1994) 'Childhood separation anxiety disorder in patients with adult anxiety disorders', *American Journal of Psychiatry*, 151(6), pp.927–9.

Livingston, R., Taylor, J.L. & Crawford, S.L. (1988) 'A study of somatic complaints and psychiatric diagnosis in children', *Journal of the American Academy of Child and Adolescent Psychiatry*, 27, pp.185–7.

Livingston, R., Nugent, H., Rader, L. & Smith, G.R. (1985) 'Family histories of depressed and severely anxious children', *American Journal of Psychiatry*, 142(12), pp.1,497–9.

Loeber, R., Green, S.M., Lahey, B.B. & Stouthamer-Loeber, M. (1989) 'Optimal informants on child disruptive behaviours', *Development and Psychopathology*, 1, pp.317–37.

Lucas, C.P. (1993) 'Diagnosis and classification of anxiety disorders in children and adolescents', *Current Opinion in Psychiatry*, 6, pp.494–9.

Macaulay, J.L. & Kleinknecht, R.A. (1989) 'Panic and panic attacks in adolescents', *Journal of Anxiety Disorders*, 3, pp.221–41.

Marks, I. (1987) 'The development of normal fear: A review', *Journal of Child Psychology and Psychiatry*, 28, pp.667–97.

Mattison, R.E. & Bagnato, S.J. (1987) 'Empirical measurement of overanxious disorder in boys 8–12 years old', *Journal of the American Academy of Child and Adolescent Psychiatry*, 26(4), pp.536–40.

McGee, R., Feehan, M., Williams, S. & Anderson, J. (1992) 'DSM-III disorders from age 11 to age 15 years', *Journal of the American Academy of Child and Adolescent Psychiatry*, 31(1), p.50.

McGee, R., Feehan, M., Williams, S., Partridge, F., Silva, P.A. & Kelly, J. (1990) 'DSM-III disorders in a large sample of adolescents', *Journal of the American Academy of Child and Adolescent Psychiatry*, 29(4), pp.611–19.

McGough, J.J., Speier, P.L. & Cantwell, D.P. (1993) 'Obsessive-compulsive disorder in childhood and adolescence', *School Psychology Review*, 22(2), pp.243–51.

Messer, S.C. & Beidel, D.C. (1994) 'Psychosocial correlates of childhood anxiety disorders', *Journal of the American Academy of Child and Adolescent Psychiatry*, 33(7), p.975.

Moreau, D. & Weissman, M.M. (1992) 'Panic disorder in children and adolescents: A review', *American Journal of Psychiatry*, 149(10), pp.1,306–14.

Mouren-Simeoni, M.C. (1992) 'A new category of anxiety disorders: Separation anxiety disorder', *Archives Françaises de Pédiatrie*, 49(1), pp.9–11.

Nelles, W.B. & Barlow, D.H. (1988) 'Do children panic?', *Clinical Psychology Review*, 8, p.359.

Ollendick, T.H., Matson, J.L. & Hersel, W.J. (1985) 'Fears in children and adolescents: Normative data', *Behaviour Research and Therapy*, 23, pp.465–7.

Ollendick, T.H., King, N.J. & Frary, R.B. (1989) 'Fears in children and adolescents: Reliability and generalizability across gender, age and nationality', *Behaviour Research and Therapy*, 27(1), pp.19–26.

Ollendick, T.H., Yule, W. & Ollier, K. (1991) 'Fears in British children and their relationship to manifest anxiety and depression', *Journal of Child Psychology and Psychiatry*, 32(2), pp.321–31.

Ollendick, T.H., Mattis, J. & King, N. (1994) 'Panic in children and adolescents: A review', *Journal of Child Psychology and Psychiatry*, 35(1), pp.113–34.

Pelcovitz, D., Kaplan, S., Goldenberg, B., Mandel, F., Lehane, J. & Guarrera, A. (1994) 'Post-traumatic stress disorder in physically abused adolescents', *Journal of the American Academy of Child and Adolescent Psychiatry*, 33(3), pp.305–12.

Perrin, S. & Last, C.G. (1992) 'Do childhood anxiety measures measure anxiety?', *Journal of Abnormal Child Psychology*, 20(6), pp.567–77.

Pliszka, S.R. (1992) 'Comorbidity of attention-deficit hyperactivity disorder and overanxious disorder', *Journal of the American Academy of Child and Adolescent Psychiatry*, 31(2), p.197.

Pollack, M.H., Otto, M.W., Rosenbaum, J.F. & Sachs, G.S. (1992) 'Personality disorders in patients with panic disorder: Association with childhood anxiety disorders, early trauma, comorbidity, and chronicity', *Comprehensive Psychiatry*, 33(2), pp.78–83.

Pollack, M.H., Otto, M.W., Hammerness, P.G. & Rosenbaum, J.F. (1993) 'Childhood anxiety in adult panic patients and their children', *Biological Psychiatry*, 33(Supplement 6A), p.42.

Popper, C.W. (1993) 'Psychopharmacologic treatment of anxiety disorders in adolescents and children', *Journal of Clinical Psychiatry*, 54(Supplement), p.52.

Pynoos, R.S., Frederick, C., Nader, K., Arroyo, W., Steinberg, A., Eth, S., Nunez, F. & Fairbanks, L. (1987) 'Life threat and post-traumatic stress in school-age children', *Archives of General Psychiatry*, 44, pp.1,057–63.

Rapee, R.M., Barrett, P.M., Dadds, M.R. & Evans, L. (1994) 'Reliability of the DSM-III-R childhood anxiety disorders using structured interview: Interrater and parent–child agreement', *Journal of the American Academy of Child and Adolescent Psychiatry*, 33(7), p.984.

Rapoport, J.L., Leonard, H.L., Swedo, S.E. & Lenane, M.C. (1993) 'Obsessive compulsive disorder in children and adolescents: Issues in management', *Journal of Clinical Psychiatry*, 54(SS), pp.27–30.

Rettew, D.C., Swedo, S.E., Leonard, H.L., Lenane, M.C. & Rapoport, J.L. (1992) 'Obsessions and compulsions across time in 79 children and adolescents with obsessive-compulsive disorder', *Journal of the American Academy of Child and Adolescent Psychiatry*, 31(6), p.1,050.

Reynolds, C.R. (1982) 'Convergent and divergent validity of the Revised Children's Manifest Anxiety Scale', *Educational and Psychological Measurement*, 42, pp.1,205–12.

Reynolds, C.R. & Paget, K.D. (1981) 'Factor analysis of the Revised Children's Manifest Anxiety Scale for blacks, whites, males and females with a national normative sample', *Journal of Consulting and Clinical Psychology*, 49(3), pp.352–9.

Reynolds, C.R. & Paget, K. (1983) 'National normative and reliability data for the Revised Children's Manifest Anxiety Scale', *School Psychology Review*, 12, pp.324–36.

Reynolds, C.R. & Richmond, B.O. (1978) ' "What I think and feel": A revised measure of children's manifest anxiety', *Journal of Abnormal Child Psychology*, 6(2), pp.271–80.

Rosenbaum, J.F., Biederman, J., Bolduc, E.A., Hirshfeld, D.R., Faraone, S.V. & Kagan, J. (1992) 'Comorbidity of parental anxiety disorders as risk for childhood-onset anxiety in inhibited children', *American Journal of Psychiatry*, 149(4), pp.475–81.

Russo, M.F. & Beidel, D.C. (1994) 'Comorbidity of childhood anxiety disorders and externalising disorders: Prevalence, associated characteristics and validation issues', *Clinical Psychology Review*, 14(3), pp.199–221.

Rutter, M., Tizard, J., Yule, W., Graham, P. & Whitmore, K. (1976) 'Research report: Isle of Wight studies, 1964–1974', *Psychological Medicine*, pp.313–32.

Ryan, N.D. (1992) 'The pharmacologic treatment of child and adolescent depression', *Pediatric Psychopharmacology*, 15(1), pp.29–39.

Ryan, N.D., Puig-Antich, J. & Ambrusini, P. et al. (1987) 'The clinical picture of major depression in children and adolescents', *Archives of General Psychiatry*, 44, pp.854–61.

Schapiro, A.K. & Schapiro, E. (1992) 'Evaluation of the reported association of obsessive-compulsive symptoms or disorder with Tourette's Disorder', *Comprehensive Psychiatry*, pp.152–65.

Scherer, M.W. & Nakamura, C.Y. (1968) 'A fear survey schedule for children (FSS-FC): A factor analytic comparison with manifest anxiety (CMAS)', *Behaviour Research and Behaviour*, 6, pp.173–82.

Schapiro, A.K., Schapiro, E.S., Young, J.G. & Feinberg, T.E. (1988) *Gilles de la Tourette Syndrome*, New York: Raven Press, p.123.

Sheehan, D.V., Sheehan, K.E. & Minichiello, W.E. (1981) 'Age of onset of phobic disorders: A reevaluation', *Comprehensive Psychiatry*, 22, pp.544–53.

Silverman, W.K. (1991) 'Diagnostic reliability of anxiety disorders in children using structured interviews', *Journal of Anxiety Disorders*, 5, p.105.

Silverman, W.K. & Eisen, A.R. (1992) 'Age differences in the reliability of parent and child reports of child anxious symptomatology using a structured interview', *Journal of the American Academy of Child and Adolescent Psychiatry*, 31(1), p.117.

Silverman, W.K. & Rabian, B. (1995) 'Test-retest reliability of the DSM-III-R childhood anxiety disorders symptoms using the Anxiety Disorders Interview Schedule for Children', *Journal of Anxiety Disorders*, 9(2), p.139.

Stavrakaki, C., Vargo, B., Boodoosingh, L. & Roberts, N. (1987a) 'The relationship between anxiety and depression in children: Rating scales and clinical variables', *Canadian Journal of Psychiatry*, 32(6), pp.433–9.

Stavrakaki, C., Vargo, B., Roberts, N. & Boodoosingh, L. (1987b) 'Concordance among sources of information for ratings anxiety and depression in children', *Journal of the American Academy of Child and Adolescent Psychiatry*, 26(5), pp.733–7.

Stevenson, J., Batten, N. & Cherner, M. (1992) 'Fears and fearfulness in children and adolescents: A genetic analysis of twin data', *Journal of Child Psychology and Psychiatry*, 33(6), pp.977–85.

Strauss, C.C. & Last, C.G. (1993) 'Social and simple phobias in children', *Journal of Anxiety Disorders*, 7(2), pp.141–52.

Strauss, C.C., Last, C.G., Hersen, M. & Kazdin, A.E. (1988a) 'Association between anxiety and depression in children and adolescents with anxiety disorders', *Journal of Abnormal Child Psychology*, 16(1), pp.57–68.

Strauss, C.C., Lease, C.A., Last, C.G. & Francis, G. (1988b) 'Overanxious disorder: An examination of developmental differences', *Journal of Abnormal Child Psychology*, 16(4), pp.433–43.

Thapar, A. & McGuffin, P. (1995) 'Are anxiety symptoms in childhood heritable?', *Journal of Child Psychology and Psychiatry*, 36(3), pp.439–47.

Thomsen, P.H. (1992) 'Obsessive-compulsive disorder in adolescence: Differential diagnostic considerations in relation to schizophrenia and BPD – A comparison of phenomenology and sociodemographic characteristics', *Psychopathology,* 25(6), pp.301–10.

Thomsen, P.H. (1993) 'Obsessive compulsive disorder in children and adolescents: Self reported obsessive compulsive behaviour in pupils in Denmark', *Acta Psychiatrica Scandinavica,* 88(3), pp.212–17.

Thomsen, P.H. (1994) 'Obsessive compulsive disorder in children and adolescents: A review of the literature', *European Child and Adolescent Psychiatry,* 3(3), pp.138–58.

Thyer, B.A. (1991) 'Diagnosis and treatment of child and adolescent anxiety disorders', *Behaviour Modification,* 15(3), p.310.

Toro, J., Cervera, M., Osejo, E. & Salamero, M. (1992) 'Obsessive-compulsive disorder in childhood and adolescence: A clinical study', *Journal of Child Psychology, Psychiatry and Allied Disciplines,* 33(6), pp.1,025–37.

Turner, S.M., Beidel, D.C. & Costello, A. (1987) 'Psychopathology in the offspring of anxiety disorders patients', *Journal of Consulting and Clinical Psychology,* 55(2), pp.229–35.

Van Winter, J.T. & Stickler, G.B. (1984) 'Panic attack syndrome', *Journal of Paediatrics,* 105, pp.661–5.

Vasey, M.W. (1993) 'Development and cognition in childhood anxiety: The example of worry', *Advances in Clinical Child Psychology,* 15, pp.1–39.

Velez, C.N., Johnson, J. & Cohen, P. (1989) 'A longitudinal analysis of selected risk factors for childhood psychopathology', *Journal of the American Academy of Child and Adolescent Psychiatry,* 28, pp.861–4.

Verhulst, F.C. & Van der Ende, J. (1992) 'Agreement between parents' reports and adolescents' self reports of problem behaviour', *Journal of Child Psychology and Psychiatry,* 33(6), pp.1,011–24.

Vila, G. (1993) 'Pharmacotherapy for anxiety disorders in children and adolescents', *Annales de Psychiatrie,* 8(1), pp.13–17.

Vitiello, B., Behar, D., Wolfson, S. & McLeer, S. (1990) 'Diagnosis of panic disorder in prepubertal children', *Journal of the American Academy of Child and Adolescent Psychiatry,* 29(5), pp.782–4.

Warren, R. & Zgourides, G. (1988) 'Panic attacks in high school students: Implications for prevention and intervention', *Phobia Practice and Research Journal,* 1, pp.97–113.

Werry, J.S. (1991) 'Overanxious disorder: A review of its taxonomic properties', *Journal of the American Academy of Child and Adolescent Psychiatry,* 30(4), pp.533–44.

Whitaker, A., Johnson, J., Shaffer, D., Rapoport, J.L., Kalikow, K., Walsh, B.T., Davies, M., Braiman, S. & Dolinsky, A. (1990) 'Uncommon troubles in young people: Prevalence estimates of selected psychiatric disorders in a nonreferred adolescent population', *Archives of General Psychiatry,* 47, pp.487–96.

Woolston, J.L., Rosenthal, S.L., Riddle, M.A., Sparrow, S.S., Cicchetti, D. & Zimmerman, L.D. (1989) 'Childhood comorbidity of anxiety/affective and behaviour disorders', *Journal of the American Academy of Child and Adolescent Psychiatry,* 28(5), pp.707–13.

Yule, W. (1992) 'Post traumatic stress disorder in children', *International Journal of Psychology,* 27(3–4), p.440.

Zeitlin, H. (1986) *The Natural History of Psychiatric Disorder in Children,* Institute of Psychiatry, Maudsley Monographs, Oxford: Oxford University Press, p.1.

Zitrin, C.M. & Ross, D.C. (1988) 'Early separation anxiety and adult agoraphobia', *Journal of Nervous and Mental Disease,* 176(10), pp.621–5.

3 Sources of anxiety

Renuka Nagraj

Anxiety is a normal and universal emotion which is essential for human functioning. It is defined as a 'tense emotional state', and is often marked by such physical symptoms as tension, tremor, sweating, palpitations and increased pulse rate. The word 'anxiety' stems from the Latin word *anxietas*, which connotes an experience of agitation, dread and uncertainty. There is also a suggestion that it had its origins in another Latin word, *angere*, which means to choke or to strangle, which is sometimes implied in the present-day connotation. While fear could be related to a specific object or situation, anxiety is non-specific, diffuse and anticipatory. Although distinctions have been made, the terms 'fear' and 'anxiety' are often used relatively interchangeably.

In children, fears and anxieties are common, usually temporary, many tending to be age- or time-specific. Developmentally, some fears are more common at some stages, starting with the startle reaction to stimuli during infancy. In infancy, sensory experiences predominate, and are major sources of fear. Young infants are afraid of loss of support, loud noises, strange objects and strange persons. By about 4 months, infants can be seen to show distress with strangers, which can be a somewhat delayed reaction, but by 7–8 months, there is a more immediate reaction of distress and unhappiness when the child is exposed to a stranger or strange situation. Children develop distress at being separated from their mother or caretaker. This separation anxiety increases until about the age of 18 months, and then slowly decreases in intensity. One-to-two-year-olds thus show a range of fears, including separation from parents and fear of strangers. These decline during pre-school years.

In pre-school years, fear of animals and insects, fear of the dark, fear of being left alone and fear of imaginary creatures emerge, which decrease during middle childhood.

Anxiety due to loss of self-esteem can be profound in middle childhood. In later childhood and during adolescence, interpersonal and social anxieties, fear of open or closed spaces and fear of school emerge. Concerns about performance (Bauer, 1980) and fears of war, health and bodily injury become more prominent.

The types of fears children experience at different ages were illustrated in a study by Bauer (1976), in which he examined the fears of 4–6, 6–8 and 10–12-year-old children: 4–6 and 6–8-year-olds were more likely to report fear of monsters, ghosts and animals; these fears were rarely mentioned by the 10–12-year-olds. Over half of these age groups acknowledged bedtime fears, and three-quarters reported bad dreams when asked specifically about bedtime fears and frightening dreams. These fears were much less reported in the 10–12-year-olds; 6–8 and 10–12-year-olds also reported fears of bodily injury and physical danger. Bauer felt that the difference in their fears reflected general developmental trends in cognition towards separation of internal representation from objective reality.

The temperament of the child, their level of understanding, their previous experience, and the degree of personal threat the future holds for them will all have an influence on whether they develop these anxieties or not.

Anxiety can spring from different sources as the child grows up, which psycho-analysts have helped us to understand. Newborn infants are totally helpless and entirely dependent on their mother, often the primary caretaker, for all their physical needs. When such needs are not met, the child becomes distressed and cries. The absence of vital supplies is thought to be the origin of the child's first experience of anxiety.

As infants grow, and develop cognitively, they become capable of forming human attachments. When the parent figure is absent, they become distressed. Fear of losing or being abandoned by the parent becomes a source of anxiety and the basis of separation anxiety.

Charlotte was an 8-year-old girl brought to the clinic, extremely clingy towards her mother, and very fearful of going to school, refusing to go for the past several months. When pushed, she would respond with crying and tantrums, threatening to hurt herself if forced to go to school. The problems had begun about a year prior to the referral. Her mother had become depressed following a bereavement in the extended family. Her father had problems with alcohol and was a somewhat peripheral figure, being absent from home for prolonged periods due to his work.

Charlotte's separation anxiety worsened gradually over the course of the year, resulting in complete school refusal. Family work addressing the above issues and planned gradual integration resulted in her attending school full-time.

During the second year of life, children have to learn to co-operate with a more powerful person: their father or mother. Anxiety can spring from shame, disapproval of others and loss of self-esteem. The development of conscience as the child grows older is a new and powerful source of anxiety. Anxiety arises from guilt stemming from the conflict between primitive impulses and the dictates of conscience.

Too much anxiety or stress at a particular stage of life has later effects on personality. When children are exposed to circumstances that arouse in them more anxiety than they can cope with, one possible psychological mechanism available to them is to give up behaviour patterns appropriate to their age and revert to behaviour that gratified them in the past. Psychological containment – the presence of someone to receive, hold and think together about the anxiety and relate it back to the child in a more manageable way – is important.

Anxiety thus occurs when there is a conflict either between inner wishes and impulses on the one hand and the external world on the other, or between inner urges and one's own conscience. When the anxiety becomes overwhelming, the individual will attempt to regain homeostasis by certain psychological processes which protect the individual from total disorganisation. These are called the 'mechanisms of defence'.

The types of defence described by Rycroft (1972) are readily seen in children and adolescents. He considers there are three basic attitudes with which we respond to threats – attack, flight or submission:

- *Attack* – the form of coping is to reduce anxiety by mastering the situation. If the child succeeds, then pride in their achievement and growth will take place, but if the reaction is out of proportion, then it may be expressed as a need to control everything and everyone. The child may become very manipulative and succeed in achieving a good deal of control within the family – for example, ensuring that the parents do not go out on their own in the evenings.

- *Flight* – this is often a normal response to threats of physical danger, or even from one's own impulses in respect to a realistic appraisal of one's own physical or psychological weaknesses. When this defence against anxiety becomes excessive or inappropriate, a person will tend to avoid situations and people that cause anxiety. A child will show phobic symptoms. Some cases of school phobia, where school bullying may be a cause, fit into this picture.

- *Submission* – a child may become too submissive or passive in situations where assertiveness or flight would be more appropriate. It is frequently seen in children who are afraid of their own aggression. A child may become overcompliant in response to angry feelings towards the parent.

Although each of these defence mechanisms would be abnormal if carried to extremes, most can be observed, at least transiently, in normal children.

Psycho-analysts have described other types of defence mechanisms. The basic mechanism is that of repression. Here, all the unacceptable wishes or impulses are repressed into the unconscious. Although unconscious, the impulse continues to strive for release, and internal tension exists.

Some of the defence mechanisms seen in children are:

- *Regression* – this is one of the commonest defence mechanisms in children. The child reverts to behaviour characteristic of an early developmental stage where there was more gratification – for example, bedwetting in a toilet-trained child in the face of anxiety over going to hospital. An older child may react to the birth of a sibling by becoming very clingy to the mother.

- *Denial* – this is also common in children. The child may behave as if the event has not occurred – for example, on sudden death of an important person in the child's family, the child may continue with normal activities without any signs of distress.

- *Displacement* – feelings and impulses are transferred from a situation or object with which they are associated to another which will cause less distress.

- *Ritualisation* – a child may develop obsessional behaviour as a relief from anxiety. For example, Jenny was an 8-year-old girl who was referred with excessive concerns about germs over the previous 18 months. This had increased to such an extent that it limited her activities and affected the quality of her life. She would wash her hands and face repeatedly, and would feel anxious about touching even her own clothes. She would cringe when her parents cuddled or touched her.

Jenny's two siblings were much older, and had left home. Her father, with whom she had a close relationship, had been posted away in his job in the Air Force. Her mother had been ill with renal problems recently. Exploration of Jenny's anxieties revealed worries about her mother's health and anger towards her father for leaving, and worries if he would return.

• *Reaction formation* – unacceptable feelings and urges are turned into their opposite. For example, 6-year-old Natasha would never get angry with her mother, even when her mother frustrated her. She was always overconcerned for her mother's welfare, and was always too helpful.

• *Projection* – in this, one's unacceptable impulses are attributed to others. A child may unrealistically consider their teacher as hostile and punitive, while feeling angry and rebellious towards the teacher, and repress these feelings.

• *Somatisation* – some children 'somatise' their anxiety – they may develop aches and pains in their abdomen or head. For example, Alan was a 10-year-old boy who was admitted to the paediatric ward following repeated episodes of very severe abdominal pain of three months' duration. He had been admitted briefly twice before, and all organic causes had been ruled out by the paediatric and surgical teams. Each time he had been discharged, his parents would bring him back within a few days, finding it extremely hard to cope with him. During these episodes, he would scream endlessly and writhe in agony, holding on to his abdomen. These episodes occurred both at home and at school, and subsequently resulted in him not attending school.

The parents had suffered severe stresses over the year. Their business had collapsed and their house had been repossessed, which affected the parental relationship. Individual work with Alan revealed anxieties about the parents' marriage breaking up, and concerns for their welfare and well-being. Family work was also initiated to address the issues. Gradual re-integration into school was established. He made a full recovery, and has been symptom-free for over a year.

When childhood anxiety is overwhelming and defensive manoeuvres are resorted to in a massive way, symptoms may develop and last, and adult behaviour may, to some extent, become maladaptive. The child's capacity to tolerate anxiety, and their choice of coping mechanisms, will inevitably influence their developing personality. The form of the child's solution and the type of defence mechanism employed will depend not only on the child's temperament and the presence of other specific stresses that the child must face at the same time, but also on the types of solution allowed by the environment.

The way in which children express their anxiety will depend on their age and developmental stage and their individual characteristics. Pre-school children will cling excessively when anxious, insecure or miserable, or when preoccupied with worries. Those children with undue general fearfulness and anxiety will often find even brief separations from their parents, especially their mother, difficult to tolerate.

School-age children aged from 5 to 12 years do not ordinarily cling. Usually, they will tend to show tension and worry throughout the day. Some others may start complaining of tummy pains or headaches, of difficulties in getting to sleep and staying asleep, and repeated nightmares may occur. They may constantly seek reassurance and become unduly dependent. Some obsessional behaviour with rituals may develop in some children as a response to anxiety. Anxious children can often become irritable and demanding.

Adolescents more often tend to express their anxiety like adults. They can appear tense and on edge, and can become fidgety and restless. Their concentration can be affected. Like younger children, they can become irritable in mood. They may show unusual concern over bodily health and bodily appearance.

Theoretical frameworks

Theories of anxiety disorders have focused mainly on internal conflicts, learned responses to external events, maladaptive cognitions and biological factors.

Psycho-analytic theories

These assume that the sources of anxiety are internal and unconscious. It was Freud's psychodynamic formulation that heralded modern theories of anxiety. Freud (1955) postulated three theories of anxiety, based on his clinical observations. The first was that anxiety arose from dammed-up instinctual (sexual) tensions which were the result of repression of these drives. He replaced this theory with a more fundamental concept, that all anxiety is due to the birth trauma. His final formulation was that there are two types of anxiety: signal anxiety, and primary or neurotic anxiety.

Signal anxiety serves a protective function by warning the subject of the approach of danger. The danger may arise from either external or internal sources such as the potential overwhelming of defences by instinctual drives.

Primary or neurotic anxiety, on the other hand, develops when the psyche is overwhelmed by an influx of stimuli which it cannot master or cope with. Individuals will experience increasing tension, anxiety or panic if they have to remain in such a situation. For example, a child's panic about the consequences of their hostility to one parent may lead them to desire to be good and to please their parents, with consequent absence of spontaneity. Freud believed that neurotic anxiety is the result of unconscious conflict between id impulses (mainly sexual and aggressive) and the constraints imposed by the ego and superego. Although such traumatic states are most frequently seen in infancy or childhood, when the ego is relatively underdeveloped, they may also arise in adults.

Melanie Klein and her colleagues made important contributions to the understanding of anxiety. Klein (1932) postulated two types of anxiety – paranoid-schizoid and depressive anxiety. She argued that aggressive (rather than libidinal) wishes were central to anxiety. From her observations of very young children, Klein believed that the child's mental life is full of representations of 'good' and 'bad' objects, which concern libidinal and aggressive wishes towards significant others in the real world. Anxiety and guilt arise out of fear that the aggressive fantasies will destroy the object (e.g. mother) and the self (through the mechanism of projection of aggression onto the object).

In the paranoid-schizoid position, the main anxiety is that the child will be destroyed by the 'bad' object, whereas when the child has reached the depressive position, anxiety springs from their own awareness of their ambivalence and the fear that their destructive impulses have destroyed or will destroy the object that they care for and depend upon. It is a state of tension between love and aggression (life and death instincts).

Neo-Freudians considered anxiety mainly in interpersonal rather than intrapsychic terms. Neo-Freudian psychological theories of childhood anxiety looked at early social relationships, mainly between the parent, especially the mother, and the child. The mother's own anxiety can be transferred or communicated directly to the child, usually serving the mother's own psychological needs (Eisenberg, 1958). Generally, mothers are described as overprotective; they may have separation anxiety issues of their own. They tend to reinforce dependency and lack of autonomy in their children.

Learning theory

This views anxiety as triggered more by specific external events than by internal conflicts. Fears are acquired through conditioning. A neutral object (the conditioned stimulus) paired with a traumatic event (the unconditioned stimulus) produces fear of the neutral object (the conditioned response). Stimuli which resemble the original stimuli also acquire fear-producing properties. Individuals then strive to avoid encountering such situations, and successful avoidance strengthens those behaviours that led to the avoidance.

Mowrer's (1960) behavioural model of anxiety demonstrates that anxiety can act as a drive, and hence is a motivational state. Anxiety (fear) is the conditioned form of the pain reaction, which has the useful function of reinforcing behaviour that tends to avoid or prevent a recurrence of the painful situation (unconditioned stimulus).

Seligman (1970) proposed the notion of 'prepared conditioning'. He postulated that humans are biologically predisposed (or prepared) to react with fear only to certain classes of dangerous objects or situations. When these objects or situations are paired with trauma, fear conditioning occurs rapidly, and this becomes very resistant to extinction.

Cognitive theories

These theories focus on the way that anxious people think about situations, where reality is continually interpreted as dangerous. Anxious people consistently overestimate both the degree of harm and the likelihood of harm, which makes them always on the look-out for signs of danger. Cognitive distortions thus prevent normal affective or behavioural responses, which can induce anxiety.

The cognitive developmental theory proposes that as children grow, they develop increasingly stable schemata of their environment and experience. These schemata play a part in regulating the child's behaviour and information processing, and if these are disrupted, they cause anxiety (Kagan et al., 1984). These anxious schemata may remain latent until triggered by stress.

Biological theories

The most widely known of these theories was originated by Eysenck (1967). He proposed that individual differences in vulnerability to anxiety were inherent. These differences led to the individual's resting level of arousal. Eysenck's theory includes two aspects: the level of cortical arousal, and the autonomic nervous system activity. Anxiety results from the interaction of individual traits of cortical arousal and autonomic reactivity with the influence of the limbic system. Those individuals who have an anxiety disorder tend to have high resting levels of cortical arousal and high autonomic nervous system reactivity.

Barlow's theory (Barlow, 1988) proposes a biological-developmental model of anxiety. The child is born with a biological vulnerability to stress. If a negative life event then occurs, it produces disruption to the individual's ongoing activity. This results in increase in stress-related arousal, which at times can be intense. At these intense levels, neurobiological activity can trigger false alarms of fear. These can produce a sense of unpredictability and uncontrollability and a negative affective state. This negative state and the associated mono-aminergic activity can produce a chronic cycle of anxious apprehension.

Neurophysiological theories

With the development of anti-anxiety agents, several neurophysiological theories of anxiety regulation have been put forward. Gray proposes that there is a neural-behavioural inhibitory system which, when activated by specific experiences, causes subjective anxiety (Gray, 1982, 1987). Other studies suggest the involvement of the brain stem, the limbic system and the pre-frontal cortex (Gorman et al., 1989). Other studies have looked at the role of neurotransmitters and suggest gamma-amino-butyric acid, seratonin and nor-epinephrine to be the neurotransmitters most closely associated with anxiety phenomena in the central nervous system. However, even if anxiety disorders have a biochemical basis, environmental experiences undoubtedly play an important role. Such disorders may develop through an interaction between biological predispositions and childhood experiences.

Ethological theories

The ethological model derives from Darwin's contribution concerning the adaptive role of the emotions in behaviour. According to this model, the experience of anxiety is seen as an adaptive, unlearned response. Bowlby (1973) suggested a Darwinian evolutionary basis for attachment behaviour: it ensures that adults protect their young. His theory of anxiety holds that the child's sense of distress during separation is perceived and experienced as anxiety. The ability of the mother to relieve the infant's anxiety or fear increases the attachment in the infant or child.

It is interesting to consider animal models of anxiety, which have been extensively studied by Suomi et al. (1981). They found that stressful life events during development produce long-term anxiety levels – for example, young rhesus monkeys separated from a primary caregiver and introduced to a group of strangers experience a 'panic-like' anxiety, followed by a long-term, chronic anxiety.

Familial patterns

Evidence is shown in a number of studies about the high prevalence of all types of anxiety disorders among the relatives of patients with panic disorder. It has been suggested that genetic factors play a part in development of anxiety disorders, especially panic disorder and agoraphobia with panic attacks.

Family systems theory

This suggests that the anxious child acquires the mother's anxiety not by modelling, as some learning theories would suggest, but through the type of communication they receive. This has been applied particularly to childhood separation anxiety.

The roles of temperament and stressful life events in the development of anxiety in children have been studied widely. Children who, in the first year of life, are rather withdrawn, quiet and slow to warm up have a predisposition to develop anxiety reactions in later childhood. Stressful life events play a role, particularly in the case of separation anxiety disorder and school phobia, where a loss such as illness or death of a significant other or a move to a new neighbourhood or school may often precede the disorder.

Conclusion

This chapter has focused on the nature and development of childhood fears and anxieties, their expression, their sources and the various mechanisms involved. The theoretical frameworks underlying anxiety disorders in children have been considered.

Purely psychological theories offer little to explain the individual differences in the development of handicapping anxiety symptoms. Other theories have attempted to look at the nature of these differences. The various theories of anxiety in children have generated differing approaches to treatment. Although our knowledge of childhood anxiety has expanded considerably since the days of Freud, there is much more that remains to be addressed.

References

Barlow, D.H. (1988) *Anxiety and its Disorders: The Nature and Treatment of Anxiety and Panic*, New York: Guilford Press.

Bauer, D. (1976) 'An exploratory study of developmental changes in children's fears', *Journal of Child Psychology and Psychiatry*, 17, pp.69–74.

Bauer, D. (1980) 'Childhood fears in developmental perspective', in Hersov, L. & Berg, I. (eds) *Out of School*, London: John Wiley, pp.189–208.

Beck, A.T. & Emery, G. (1985) *Anxiety Disorders and Phobias: A Cognitive Perspective*, New York: Basic Books.

Bowlby, J. (1973) *Attachment and Loss, Vol.2: Separation, Anxiety and Anger*, New York: Basic Books.

Eisenberg, L. (1958) 'School phobia: A study in the communication of anxiety', *American Journal of Psychiatry*, 114, pp.712–18.

Eysenck, H.J. (1967) *The Biological Basis of Personality*, Springfield, IL: Charles C. Thomas.

Freud, S. (1955) 'Inhibitions, symptoms and anxiety', in Strachey, J. (ed.) *The Standard Edition of the Complete Psychological Works of Sigmund Freud*, Vol.XX: 1926, London: Hogarth Press, pp.75–174.

Gittelman, R. (ed.) (1986) *Anxiety Disorders of Childhood*, New York: Guilford Press.

Gorman, J.M., Liebowitz, M.R., Fyer, A.J. & Stein, J. (1989) 'A neuroanatomical hypothesis for panic disorder', *American Journal of Psychiatry*, 146, pp.148–61.

Gray, J.A. (1982) *The Neuropsychology of Anxiety: An Enquiry into the Functions of the Septo-hippocampal System*, Oxford: Oxford University Press.

Gray, J.A. (1987) *The Psychology of Fear and Stress* (2nd edn), Cambridge: Cambridge University Press.

Kagan, J. (1988) 'Biological basis of childhood shyness', *Science*, 240, pp.167–71.

Kagan, J., Reznick, J.S., Clarke, C. & Snidman, N. (1984) 'Behavioural inhibition to the unfamiliar', *Child Development*, 55, pp.2,212–25.

Klein, M. (1932) *The Psychoanalysis of Children*, London: Hogarth.

Klein, R.G. & Last, C.G. (1989) *Anxiety Disorders in Children*, Newbury Park, CA: Sage Publications.

Mowrer, O.H. (1960) *Learning Theory and Behaviour*, New York: John Wiley.

Rycroft, C. (1972) *Anxiety Neuroses*, London: Penguin.

Seligman, M. (1970) 'On the generality of the laws of learning', *Psychological Review*, 77, pp.406–18.

Suomi, S.J. (1986) 'Anxiety-like disorders in young nonhuman primates', in Gittelman, R. (ed.) *Anxiety Disorders of Childhood*, New York: Guilford Press, pp.1–23.

Suomi, S.J., Kraemer, G.W., Baysinger, C.M., et al. (1981) 'Inherited and experiential factors associated with individual differences in anxious behaviour displayed by rhesus monkeys', in Klein, D.F. & Rabkin, J. (eds) *Anxiety: New Research and Changing Concepts*, New York: Raven Press, pp.179–99.

4 Assessment, with a view to treatment planning

Anthony Roberts

General considerations

There are a number of important considerations that must be borne in mind when approaching the issue of assessment of a child or adolescent with an anxiety-related problem. In some instances, the issues are similar to those which apply to adults; in some instances, there are important differences.

Developmental issues: The need for a multimodal assessment

Kendall et al. (1991) note that the assessment process must address the extensive developmental changes that are occurring during childhood. As a simplification, these changes within the individual may be categorised as cognitive, emotional and biological. The different cognitive developmental stages determine how we interview the child, and how we make sense of what the child says to us (see Bierman, 1984, for a detailed review, including suggestions of interviewing techniques to match the child's understanding).

Age and developmental stage also determine norms. This applies particularly to fears: for example, fear of the dark at the age of 4 would not be unusual; the same fear at the age of 10 would be considered abnormal (see King et al., 1988, for a detailed account of the prevalence of various fears). On the other hand, some symptoms are not normal at any age – for example, severe anxiety associated with obsessions, or symptomatology associated with panic attacks.

51

Situational specificity and observer bias

Achenbach et al. (1987), in a detailed meta-analysis of studies on behavioural and emotional problems of children and adolescents, note the considerable variations in reports by different informants.

Thus the child's behaviour (including verbal behaviour) will be influenced by the context, including the relationship with the interviewer. This means that, where possible, we must aim for a multimodal assessment, with information on all three channels (cognitive, behavioural, physiological) from as many informants and about as many situations as possible.

Diagnosis: From DSM-III-R to DSM-IV

Much of the literature on anxiety disorders in children and adolescents relates to DSM-III-R. DSM-IV (American Psychiatric Association, 1994) contains important differences compared to DSM-III-R. For example, of the three original categories under 'anxiety disorders of childhood' – separation anxiety disorder, avoidant disorder of childhood and adolescence, and overanxious disorder – only the first remains in DSM-IV as an anxiety disorder specific to childhood. The criteria of the remaining two are subsumed under 'adult anxiety disorders'. For a detailed review of the differences between DSM-III-R and DSM-IV criteria, see Clark et al. (1994).

Comorbidity: A single diagnosis may be insufficient

When assessing a child with an anxiety disorder, the clinician needs to be hypervigilant with respect to the presence of comorbidity. Studies of school phobics indicate a degree of comorbidity with affective disorder, anxiety disorder and conduct disorder (Bernstein & Garfinkel, 1986; Bernstein et al., 1990). In a study of 988 female adolescents (Bernstein et al., 1989), those reporting high anxiety also reported increased incidence of physical and sexual abuse, somatic complaints, poor school performance, use of street drugs, and a family history related to depression. Clark et al. (1994) note that while studies suggest that depressive disorders are the most common comorbid disorders associated with anxiety disorders in adolescents, important associations may also exist between alcohol disorders and disruptive behaviour disorders. The authors also note that multiple anxiety disorders are common in adolescents sampled from the community. For a recent, detailed review of comorbidity in relation to DSM-III-R and DSM-IV, see Kendall and Brady (1995).

Of related importance is the fact that DSM-III-R disorders are not equally distributed across the population. Kessler et al. (1994) present important findings from their National Comorbidity Survey. In a sample with an age range of 15–54 years, nearly 50% of respondents reported at least one lifetime DSM-III-R disorder. The most common disorders were major depressive episode, alcohol dependence, social phobia and simple phobias. Furthermore, more than half of all the lifetime disorders occurred in the 14% of the population who had a history of three or more comorbid disorders. This 14% also included the majority of people with severe disorders.

While it would be dangerous to assume that such a pattern applies to children and adolescents, such findings should put us on our guard when considering a single diagnosis.

Has the child been abused? The issue of trauma in childhood

Symptoms of anxiety presenting in childhood, adolescence and adulthood can be a component of the post-traumatic response (Horowitz et al., 1979; Pynoos et al., 1987; Pynoos, 1990; Yule & Udwin, 1991; Scott & Stradling, 1992; Walker et al., 1992; Schwartz & Perry, 1994). While the influence of disasters will usually be elicited in a history, the existence of previous (and often ongoing) child abuse in its various manifestations may not be so easily demonstrated. Again, the clinician's suspicion should be aroused where an anxiety disorder is diagnosed but where the formulation is incomplete because of a lack of disclosed aetiology.

The dilemma of varying therapist conceptual frameworks

One of the dilemmas facing the clinician is that of the varying conceptual frameworks that may be used to understand the young person and their problems.

For some, anxiety may be viewed in the context of interpersonal processes and family systems. For others, anxiety may be conceptualised in psychodynamic, cognitive or behavioural terms.

Few, if any, clinicians have developed a 'theory of everything', superordinate to all previous theories. When assessing patients, clinicians need to be aware that their framework is inevitably incomplete, and is in itself a belief system, more or less consistent with the available evidence, and more or less in sympathy with current paradigms concerning mental health.

In addition to the effects of transference and counter-transference, the therapist's conceptual framework will also affect the way in which the therapist views both the young person's symptoms and the young person themself. In turn, such views will also affect the relationship between the therapist and the young person. They may also alter the therapist's expectations regarding therapy and therapeutic outcome. Thus, a young person conceptualised as having a 'personality disorder', or being a 'drug addict', may be viewed in a very different way from someone seen as being caught up in a web of family pathology, or being the victim of psychic trauma such as child abuse.

The need for an assessment process

There are several purposes of the assessment process:

- to establish rapport with the child and their family;
- to arrive at a diagnosis or diagnoses, to exclude differential diagnoses and to consider the possibility of comorbid conditions;
- to ascertain which areas (if any) require further detailed and specialist investigations;
- to arrive at a provisional formulation, with a view to treatment planning;
- to evaluate the success of a treatment package.

The initial stages of the assessment process will involve a detailed history. For a more detailed account of the history-taking process, see Graham (1991); King et al. (1988) and Ollendick (1995). In many cases, particularly those involving younger children, the interview will have a number of therapist agendas; as well as being involved in a behavioural or cognitive behavioural analysis of the child's problems, the therapist will be taking a family history and also observing the family interactions and dynamics. There may also be information regarding psychiatric disorder in other family members.

At this stage, we will move on to the detailed history, with its various components.

The history

The referral

Whose idea was it to come to the clinic?

What was the reaction to the referral?

Who wanted to come, and who did not?

Note the importance of ascertaining who in the family feels that there is a problem. These questions frequently reveal splits within the family, or disagreements between family members and the referrer. Frequently, families are 'sent' to clinicians, often by professionals who feel that the child needs help, but where neither the parents nor the child see any such need.

The problem – the family's view

The view of various family members, including the young person

What do the family see the problem as being?

It is necessary to establish a preliminary view of the family members' constructs about the problem:

Who first noticed the problem?

Who is most worried about the problem?

Here we have the opportunity to flush out the anxieties that other members of the family have concerning the child and their problem – anxieties that indeed may be greater than the child's own anxieties. This may be relevant later, in connection with the aetiology.

How is it a problem?

We can see the way in which the referred problems of the identified patient impinge on the rest of the family. A socially phobic child may, for example, prevent their family participating in normal family outings; such behaviour might be an indicator of hierarchy problems within the family. In some cases, there will be collusion, as when, for example, a family member collaborates in a child's compulsions. In other cases, the problem may provide secondary gain for a family member, as when a fearful child comes into their parents' bed, or a school-phobic child remains at home with their mother.

What changes would the family like to happen as a result of coming for help?

- to uncover areas of agreement or disagreement as to the goals of treatment;
- to make the first steps towards establishing goals of treatment.

Why have the family come at this point of time?

This may be straightforward, for example in anticipation of problems in a new school; it may be less straightforward, for example when the family arrive for help in order to preempt a prosecution for school non-attendance. The child's presentation may be a 'ticket' for the discussion of other problems.

How does the family explain the problem/behaviour?

This provides a further opportunity to observe the family's constructs. It may help predict implications for treatment, as when, for example, the child's school is blamed for the existence of the child's anxiety state.

Having looked at the circumstances surrounding the problem, we can now proceed to look in more detail at the problem itself.

The problem itself

What is the precise nature of the problem or symptoms?

What is the duration of the symptoms?

Were there any precipitants?

See Ollendick and King (1991), who explore Rachman's (1977) theory of 'three pathways of fear' – direct conditioning, modelling, and instruction/information – in relation to children and adolescents. All three pathways were found to be relevant to the ten most common children's fears. Therefore it may be relevant to consider:

Have there been any personal frightening experiences?

Is there any family member (or other relevant adult or child) who provides a role model for anxiety?

Look also for a parent's idiosyncratic, dysfunctional or contextually unhelpful belief system, such as a belief in ghosts, or overestimation of the risk of a natural disaster. It can also include a parent's anxiety about the identified patient. Parental anxiety about, for example, fire may be expressed in compulsive checking behaviour. See reference to comorbidity of anxiety disorder on p.52.

Has there been any information/instruction?

Look for direct instruction, in the form of information (including mis-information), from peers or adults ('cows bite', 'monsters will climb out of the toilet'). Consider also the possible impact of specific frightening TV news programmes or plays (e.g. scenes depicting war, violence, disaster, illness, ghosts or poltergeists) or unsuitable or frightening videotapes.

How often does the problem manifest itself?

Have there been any remissions or exacerbations?

The above may give further clues to the possible aetiology of the problem, and pointers to treatment.

How severe is the problem?

How well does the child function?

What is the degree of handicap?

See Axis V of DSM-IV for discussion of global assessment of functioning. Can the child function in the major areas of school, family life or peer group relationships?

Is the problem episodic, or is it present all the time?

Is there persistent worrying, as in generalised anxiety disorder, or is the problem episodic and paroxysmal, as in panic attacks?

What is the state of the patient between attacks?

Outside the anxiety-provoking situation, the patient may be asymptomatic.

Detailed description of the problem – an interactional model

Padesky (1986) describes a general model (see Figure 4.1) which assumes a degree of coupling between emotion, behaviour, physiology, cognition

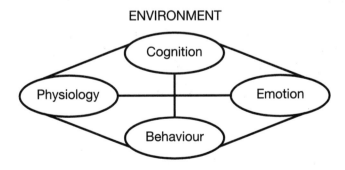

ENVIRONMENT

Cognition

Physiology

Emotion

Behaviour

Figure 4.1   Padesky's five-component cognitive behavioural model (Copyright © C.A. Padesky, 1986)

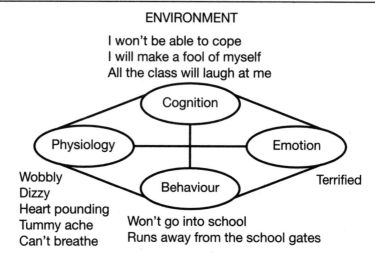

Figure 4.2   School refusal: Annotation as a joint exercise with the young person

and environment. This model is a useful *aide-mémoire* when considering the components of a problem, and is straightforward enough to be shared with the child and their family. The clinician might, for example, when discussing the symptoms and signs of the child's anxiety disorder, annotate the basic model as a collaborative exercise, as in Figure 4.2.

Using this model as an adjunct, the clinician can enquire about the four components of the presenting anxiety in addition to environmental influences. For a detailed cognitive behavioural assessment schedule, see Kirk (1989).

Cognitions

Does the child have habitual thoughts or worries which are associated with fear or anxiety?
For example, the clinician might ask:

When this frightening thing happened, what thoughts were going through your head?

What were you afraid might happen?

What is the worst that could happen?

The anxious child has a tendency to ask 'What if . . . ' Look for catastrophic thoughts, for example that a parent may not be at home when the child returns, that the parent might meet with a road traffic accident, or that the whole class might laugh when the child goes into school. See Ronan et al. (1994) for details of questionnaires which tap these negative cognitions. Included here also are the obsessional thoughts reported in patients with obsessive-compulsive disorder. See Salkovskis and Kirk (1989) for a detailed account of the principal content of obsessions. Consider also the 'neutralising' (i.e. anxiety-reducing) cognitions frequently engaged in by patients with obsessive-compulsive disorder.

Does the patient experience imagery and/or flashbacks?

Visual imagery frequently plays an important role in the maintenance of anxiety disorders. Look for intrusive imagery in post-traumatic stress disorder and child abuse (including child sexual abuse).

To what extent are the cognitions or images voluntary?

Are there attempts at cognitive avoidance?

Patients may attempt to avoid talking about difficult issues in the session; alternatively, they may report that they have attempted to suppress unwelcome thoughts or images, such as occur in obsessive-compulsive disorder or post-traumatic stress disorder.

Emotion

When this happened, how did it leave you feeling?

How did you feel inside?

It can be misleading to assume the emotion that the young person is experiencing. Emotions reported may not only be anxiety and/or fear, but dread, sadness, guilt, revulsion, anger or hatred, according to the situation.

Physiology: The occurrence of somatic symptoms and signs

- palpitations?
- sweating?
- trembling or shaking?
- nausea?
- feeling of 'butterflies'?
- feeling of choking, unable to breathe?
- chest pain or discomfort?

- numbness, 'pins and needles', tingling?
- chills or hot flushes?

These symptoms of anxiety may be either observed by others, for example parents, or experienced by the patient, or both. The Beck Anxiety Inventory (see pp.66–7) provides a useful checklist of symptoms of somatic anxiety for older children.

Secondary problems may occur when such symptoms are interpreted by the patient as implying physical or mental illness.

Behaviour

How does the child behave when they are anxious?

Have there been any attempts to confront the anxiety?

Does the young person show avoidance behaviour?

If so:

Does the young person attempt to leave the anxiety-provoking situation (active avoidance)?

Does the young person avoid the anxiety-provoking situation in the first place (passive avoidance)?

Is there evidence of anxiety-neutralising behaviour, as in the compulsions of obsessive-compulsive disorder?

Also look for attempts to avoid situations where obsessions might be triggered, and avoidance of situations which might trigger imagery in post-traumatic stress disorder.

Is there evidence of substance misuse?

The young person may abuse drugs, alcohol or solvents in an attempt to avoid unpleasant thoughts or emotions.

Does the young person seek reassurance?

Does the young person receive reassurance?

Frequently, a parent will unwittingly collude in this form of avoidance – the avoidance of uncertainty.

Modulating variables

What are the variables affecting the problem?

Which of them cause the problem to be worse, or better?

The problem may also be affected by physiology, for example it may be worse when the patient is tired.

Are the young person's problems and behaviour better or worse in the presence of one or other parent, or both, or neither?

Consider the possibility of covert reinforcement of anxious or avoidant behaviour by a parent. Alternatively, a parent may provide an anxious role model at the time that the problem is occurring, for example when a phobic child reaches the school gates. Disagreement between parents may provide the child with contradictory messages.

Is the problem affected by the presence of others – for example, peers?

Is the extent of anxious behaviour different at home compared to school?

What are the consequences of anxiety-related behaviour for the child?

What are the consequences for the family?

Family preoccupation with the problem may mask other family problems, as when, for example, the child consistently comes into the parents' bed (masking marital problems) or the school-phobic child remains at home as a companion to a housebound parent.

Look for reciprocal influence, where the behaviour of both the child and the parent each rewards the other in a maladaptive fashion (see Bandura, 1969).

Family

Family composition

- parents?
- step-parents?
- aunts and uncles?
- grandparents?

Relatives outside the immediate nuclear family may often be able to take a more detached view of the young person's problem.

Medical or psychiatric history within the family

- occupations, where applicable?
- previous medical history?
- previous psychiatric history?
- current physical and mental health?

The young person may have unacknowledged worries about a parent's mental health as well as their physical health. It is not uncommon for a young person to be anxious lest a parent engage in deliberate self-harm.

A number of studies show increased psychiatric morbidity in families of probands with anxiety disorders (Bernstein & Borchardt, 1990; Bernstein & Garfinkel, 1988; Bernstein et al., 1990; Deltito & Hahn, 1993; Fyer, 1993). For a brief but useful summary of familial clustering, see American Psychiatric Association (1994) under the headings for each disorder.

Accommodation

In addition to quality of accommodation, consider security of tenure and possible financial problems in relation to mortgage.

What are the sleeping arrangements?

Look for cross-generational sleeping arrangements as evidence of possible family dysfunction, including enmeshment, overprotectiveness or marital problems.

What is the neighbourhood like?

In violent or socially-deprived neighbourhoods, the fears may indeed be realistic. However, this does not exclude the young person receiving a formal diagnosis of an anxiety disorder, and the family response may be dysfunctional.

The young person

Personal and developmental history of the young person

- pregnancy?
- birth?
- perinatal circumstances?
- early mother–child relationship?
- temperamental characteristics?
- developmental milestones?

- past medical history?
- past psychiatric history?
- contact with child guidance or child psychiatry departments?

- periods spent away from home:
  - hospitalisations?
  - accommodation by fosterparents or social services?

- Major life events for the young person and their family?

School and outside interests

- schools attended?
- current school?
- academic progress?
- favourite subjects?
- relationships with peers?
- school societies, clubs, etc.?
- ambition on leaving school?
- hobbies and interests at home?
- favourite TV programmes?
- favourite pop groups?
- activities with friends?

When discussing school and leisure activities, the therapist has an opportunity to assess the child's strengths; by focusing on those activities where the child shows strengths, the therapist has an opportunity to simultaneously engage the child and enhance the child's self-esteem.

Psychosocial development

Does the young person have friends?

Are they friends of the same or the opposite sex?

Are they of similar age?

Does the young person have a particular close friend to whom to turn?

Does the young person have a boyfriend or a girlfriend?

Are they sexually active?

Is the young person appropriately assertive?

Here the clinician can obtain further evidence of the degree of accomplishment of age-appropriate maturational tasks, thus enhancing the description of the psychosocial backdrop against which the problem may be viewed.

Observation of the young person and their family

Even when the presentation is that of an older adolescent, who may wish to be seen alone, it can be helpful to observe family interactions.

Assessment of family

Do all members of the family appear physically and mentally well?

There is increased morbidity among first-degree relatives of young people with anxiety disorders. Look especially for evidence of anxiety disorders and depressive disorders.

Did all the family members arrive for the interview? What was the reason given for any absences?

How do the family appear to be relating to each other?

Do the family relate warmly?

Is there evidence of marital tensions?

If the child is obviously distressed, do the family members show concern? Do any of them also become distressed?

Does any family member appear to be doing all the talking?

Is the child allowed to speak for themselves?

Look for parental overinvolvement, overprotection, lack of boundaries, enmeshment.

Does any family member appear to be scapegoated, rejected by others?

Assessment of the young person (see Eminson, 1993)

Assess the child's appearance:

Does the child appear physically well?

Are there any odd movements or mannerisms?

How does the child relate to the clinician?

Is there rapport?

Is there eye contact?

Does the child have insight into the problem?

Assess the child's mood:

Does the child present as happy, sad, angry, anxious, or exhibit other emotions?

Does the child show physiological evidence of anxiety – for example, sweating, pallor?

Speech and thought:

Is it developmentally appropriate?

Is there any evidence of psychosis, delusions or hallucinations?

Assessment instruments

There are a confusing number of assessment instruments available to the clinician, and space does not permit a description of all but a few of them. For a detailed critical review, see Chapter 5. For other reviews, see also Barrios et al. (1981), Bernstein & Borchardt (1990), Kendall (1994), Kendall et al. (1991), Kendall et al. (1992), Kendall et al. (1981), Kendall and Ronan (1990a), King et al. (1988), Ollendick (1995) and Stallings and March (1995).

We shall consider briefly three categories of instruments: structured clinical interviews, self-report scales, and parent and teacher rating scales.

Structured and semistructured clinical interviews

The Anxiety Disorders Interview Schedule for Parent and Child (ADIS-P&C) The original ADIS-C and ADIS-P (Silverman, 1987) are semi-structured interviews for children and parents which rely on DSM-III-R criteria for assessing anxiety disorders. A new structured interview based on DSM-IV (Silverman & Albano) is in press. These interviews, the ADIS-P&C, are planned to be an in-depth diagnostic tool which assesses in detail the major Axis I emotional disorders, and is worded to be used with children of all ages.

Self-report scales

Scales that measure fear, anxiety or depression

The Revised Fear Survey Schedule for Children, FSSC-R (Ollendick, 1983) Designed to access common, specific fears, this scale contains 80 items, to which the child may respond according to a three-point scale ('None', 'Some', 'A Lot'). Factor analysis has revealed a five-factor solution, the factors being 'fear of failure and criticism', 'fear of the unknown', 'fear of injury and small animals', 'fear of danger and death' and 'medical fears'. See King et al. (1991) and Ollendick et al. (1991) for the relationship between the FSSC-R and the RCMAS (see below) and Ollendick et al. (1989) for normative data on the FSSC-R.

The Revised Children's Manifest Anxiety Scale (RCMAS) (Reynolds & Richmond, 1978)   This scale, entitled 'What I think and feel', is a 37-item questionnaire, with a 'Yes/No' response to each item. In addition to the nine lie items (items designed to measure the truthfulness of the subject; see p. 86 for more details), the remaining 28 items exhibit a factor structure consisting of three clusters: (a) physiological symptoms, (b) worry/oversensitivity and (c) concentration.

The Children's Depression Inventory (CDI)   See Kovacs (1981) for a general survey of rating scales designed to assess depression in school-age children, together with discussion of the development of the CDI. The scale itself consists of 27 items, each consisting of three statements, from which the child chooses one.

The State-Trait Anxiety Inventory for Children (STAIC) (Spielberger et al., 1970)   The STAIC was designed to measure anxiety in 9–12-year-old children, but may also be used with younger or older children if their developmental stage is taken into account. There are two parts to the inventory: the 20-item A-State scale, which measures anxiety at a particular moment in time, and the A-Trait scale, which measures relatively permanent personality characteristics of anxiety-proneness. The manual contains normative data (including useful percentile ranks for various scores) for both state and trait scores, for fourth-, fifth- and sixth-grade American schoolchildren.

Dimensions of Depression for Children and Adolescents: 'What is true for me' (Harter & Nowakowski, 1987)   This is a 30-item scale for which normative data were originally obtained for American elementary and middle-school students. Each item has a total of four response choices. Results are measured on five subscales: (a) mood/affect, (b) self-worth, (c) energy/interest, (d) self-blame and (e) suicidal ideation.

The Beck Depression Inventory (BDI) (Beck et al., 1961)   The BDI consists of 21 questions covering various cognitive, behavioural and somatic symptoms of depression. For each item, there is a choice of one of four statements, rating 0–3, giving a maximum total score of 63. It is designed for use by adolescents and adults from age 13, and may be used sequentially to monitor progress in therapy from week to week.

The Beck Anxiety Inventory (BAI)   The BAI consists of 21 items which access various symptoms of anxiety, which are rated on a 0–3 scale. While designed for adolescents aged 17 and over, it may be used for younger adolescents to track the changes in symptoms of somatic anxiety during the course of therapy. The wording is simple and straightforward.

The Negative Affectivity Self-statement Questionnaire (NASSQ) (Ronan et al., 1994)   The two questionnaires, respectively for 7–10-year-olds and for 11–15-year-olds, are headed 'Thoughts about myself and others'. Both consist of statements associated with negative affect (chiefly anxiety and depression). The young person is asked to rate (on a five-point scale) how often they have had similar thoughts 'pop' into their head in the previous week.

This promises to prove a useful questionnaire for accessing the cognitive component of anxiety or depression and monitoring its variation during the course of therapy.

Multidimensional Anxiety Scale for Children (MASC) (March et al., forthcoming a, b; Parker et al., forthcoming)   This scale consists of 45 items, each rated on a four-point scale. Major factors include physical anxiety, harm avoidance, social anxiety and separation anxiety. These factors, in turn, separate into various subfactors.

Scales which measure self-concept

The Self-perception Profile for Children (Harter, 1985)   This 36-item scale accesses six domains of self-concept: (a) scholastic competence, (b) social acceptance, (c) athletic competence, (d) physical appearance, (e) behavioural conduct and (f) global self-worth. Normative data are provided for American schoolchildren from the third to eighth grades.

The Self-perception Profile for Adolescents (Harter, 1988)   This 45-item scale assesses nine domains of self-concept: (a) scholastic competence, (b) athletic competence, (c) job competence, (d) close friendship, (e) social acceptance, (f) romantic appeal, (g) physical appearance, (h) behavioural conduct and (i) global self-worth. Normative data are provided for eighth to eleventh grades.

Specialised scales

The Impact of Event Scale (Horowitz et al., 1979)   For use in patients with post-traumatic stress disorder, this is a 15-question scale which measures: (a) the degree of intrusion of memories or images of the traumatic event, and (b) the degree of avoidance of images and memories, together with emotional numbing. The scale has been successfully used with children as young as 10 (Yule & Udwin, 1991).

Parent and teacher rating scales

The Connors Rating Scales (CRS)   The Connors Parent Rating Scale (CPRS) and the Connors Teacher Rating Scale (CTRS) are currently undergoing major revision and national norming. A large number of studies have been carried out on the various forms of the original scales. The subscales include various factors such as 'hyperactive', 'conduct', 'excitable', 'anxious' and 'obsessive-compulsive'. One of the goals of the revision is to increase the number of items available for the internalising scales (see Connors, 1994).

Multi-axial assessment

Much of the literature, particularly that concerning cognitive behavioural approaches, uses DSM-IV criteria. It is for this reason, together with the existence of the comprehensive DSM-IV manual (American Psychiatric Association, 1994), that DSM-IV has been used in this chapter, rather than ICD-10.

A useful start for the clinician might be to arrive at a clinical provisional coding of information on the five axes of DSM-IV. For a detailed discussion of the value of a multi-axial classification, see LaBruzza and Mendez-Villarrubia (1994).

The DSM-IV multi-axial assessment is only the first stage in developing an overall formulation, and a useful preliminary on the road to providing a full formulation and treatment plan.

The fact that we are considering a DSM-IV diagnosis does not mean that we can ignore contextual and systemic aspects of the problem. It is merely useful at this stage to have a phenomenological description of the problem and condition, in order both to avoid major diagnostic blunders and to have a means of communication with other professionals. In addition, the provision of a clear DSM-IV diagnosis can have important implications for claims upon medical insurance, compensation claims (e.g. following child abuse) and forensic reports.

The description given below is merely a brief overview of the main anxiety disorders, together with their principal differential diagnoses. The reader is recommended to consult the DSM-IV manual for a detailed description of the individual disorders, as well as details on how to code on the other four axes.

DSM-IV disorders are coded on five axes:

- Axis I: clinical disorders;
- Axis II: personality disorders and mental retardation;
- Axis III: general medical conditions;

- Axis IV: psychosocial and environmental problems;
- Axis V: global assessment of functioning.

Axis I: Clinical disorders

The ICD classification number is given in parentheses after the name of the disorder.

The anxiety disorders

Disorders of infancy, childhood or adolescence

- Separation anxiety disorder (F93.0): look for evidence of excessive fear associated with separation from parents, in a child or adolescent under 18 (can be associated with e.g. school refusal, fear of harm to parents).

Anxiety disorders

- Panic attacks: look for sudden onset of intense fear (e.g. of dying, going mad, or losing control). Associated with symptoms of somatic anxiety, and catastrophic misinterpretation of bodily sensations.
- Agoraphobia: look for anxiety about being in places or situations where a panic attack might occur (e.g. in shopping malls, in the street, etc.).
- Panic disorder without agoraphobia (F41.0).
- Panic disorder with agoraphobia (F41.01).
- Agoraphobia without history of panic disorder (F40.00).
- Specific phobia (F40.2): look for fear or anxiety evoked by a specific object or situation (e.g. spiders, heights, flying, blood, medical situations).
- Social phobia (F40.1): look for fear of embarrassment or humiliation in social situations, fear of negative evaluation by others.
- Obsessive-compulsive disorder (F42.8): look for anxiety in association with unwanted, intrusive thoughts; attempts to neutralise by compulsive acts, which may be overt (e.g. handwashing) or mental (e.g. counting).
- Post-traumatic stress disorder (F43.1): look for history of a traumatic event; distressing recollections of the event in the form of intrusive memories, dreams, flashbacks; avoidance of stimuli associated with the traumatic event; numbing of general responsiveness – sense of alienation from others, foreshortening of future expectations.

- Acute stress disorder (F43.0): look for traumatic event within the preceding month; overlap of symptoms with post-traumatic stress disorder.
- Generalised anxiety disorder (F41.1): look for global worry, consisting of persistent anxiety or worry in a number of areas; cannot be narrowed down to specific areas as in social phobia, simple phobia, agoraphobia, separation anxiety disorder.
- Anxiety disorder due to a general medical condition (F06.4): see DSM-IV manual for details of a number of medical conditions that can *per se* give rise to symptoms of anxiety.
- Substance-induced anxiety disorder: look for symptoms of anxiety related either to intoxication with or withdrawal from drugs (e.g. withdrawal from benzodiazepines).

The principal differential diagnoses

Disorders usually first diagnosed in infancy, childhood or adolescence

Tic disorders

- Tourette's disorder (F95.2).
- Chronic motor or vocal tic disorder (F95.1).
- Transient tic disorder (F95.0).

In all the three disorders listed above, look for movements which are less complex than rituals in obsessive-compulsive disorder, and are not an attempt to neutralise an obsession.

Delirium, dementia, amnesic and other cognitive disorders

- Delirium (F05.0): look for a short time course with no known stressors; disturbances in consciousness, cognition, perception. May involve hallucinations. Presence of a physical illness may not be immediately obvious, as in certain forms of encephalitis.

Psychotic disorders

- Schizophrenia (F20.xx).
- Delusional disorder (F22.0).
- Brief psychotic disorder (F23.xx).
- Psychotic disorder due to a general medical condition (F06.x).
- Substance-induced psychotic disorder.

In all the five disorders listed above, look for anxiety related to delusions (e.g. of being persecuted; having a physical illness) and anxiety related to hallucinations.

Mood disorders

- Major depressive disorder (F32.x): look for depressed mood; loss of usual interests; sleep disturbance; feelings of worthlessness, suicidal ideation; fatigue; loss of energy. May mimic social phobia if patient stays indoors through fatigue or lack of interest.

Somatoform disorders

- Somatisation disorder (F45.0): look for history of multiple physical symptoms, affecting various sites and organ systems. Focus of anxiety or worry, however, is limited to the physical symptoms, in contradistinction to generalised anxiety disorder.
- Hypochondriasis (F45.2): look for anxiety or fear related to pre-occupation that one has a serious physical illness; continued mis-interpretation of symptoms, despite medical reassurance.
- Body dysmorphic disorder (F45.2): look for excessive anxiety or preoccupation in relation to imagined body defect and personal appearance. Excludes anxiety about body image in relation to anorexia nervosa.

Eating disorders

- Anorexia nervosa (F50.0): main anxiety or fear (if present) is that of gaining weight, in addition to other criteria for anorexia nervosa.

Other disorders

- Trichotillomania (F63.3): look for recurrent pulling out of one's hair, with tension preceding the act, and relief after it. Unlike obsessive-compulsive disorder, obsessional thoughts are absent.
- Adjustment disorder (F43.xx): look for a stressor (other than be-reavement) preceding development of problems. Symptoms even-tually disappear following removal of the stressor.
- Stereotypic movement disorder (F98.4): look for repetitive motor behaviour. Generally less complex movements than the compulsive rituals seen in obsessive-compulsive disorder.
- Avoidant personality disorder (F60.6): look for anxiety or fear in most social situations. Alternative conceptualisation to social phobia, generalised.

- Schizoid personality disorder (F60.1): look for lack of interest in relating to others. Detachment and indifference, compared to the anxiety manifest in social phobia.

Axis II: Personality disorders and mental retardation

These are mentioned here for the sake of completeness. The clinician might wish to be wary of using the term 'personality disorder' in children and adolescents.

Axis III: General medical conditions

There are a number of ways in which general medical conditions are relevant. In some cases, the medical condition may be relevant to the aetiology or worsening of the condition. In others, an anxiety state may be a reaction to an illness that is perceived as life-threatening or incapacitating. In other instances, there may be pharmacological implications (e.g. medical conditions preventing the use of chosen psychotropic drugs).

Axis IV: Psychosocial and environmental problems

This axis is likely to be of particular importance when considering children and adolescents. DSM-IV groups these problems into the following categories:

1 Problems with the primary support group: look for major life events within the family (e.g. births, marriages, deaths, remarriage, serious illness); child neglect and abuse, removal of the child from the home; abnormal parenting; death or illness of animals.
2 Problems related to the social environment: look for e.g. death or loss of friend; racial discrimination; problems with neighbours; isolation of adolescents in rural communities.
3 Educational problems: look for discordant relationships with teachers and peers, as well as academic difficulties.
4 Occupational problems.
5 Housing problems: look for inadequate housing; threatened or recent eviction; homelessness; unsafe or otherwise unsatisfactory neighbourhood; disputes with neighbours.
6 Economic problems: unemployment; poverty; threat of repossession of home.
7 Problems with access to healthcare services: look for inadequate or inaccessible healthcare services for patient or their family; inadequate health insurance.

8 Problems related to interaction with the legal system: look for young person arrested, imprisoned, victim of crime; ongoing litigation against the patient, or on behalf of the patient (e.g. for compensation); when patient is the victim of child abuse, interviews by the police or social services; appearance in court as a witness.

9 Other psychosocial or environmental problems: look for exposure to psychic trauma outside the home – war, disasters or other forms of traumatic stress; discord with professionals.

Axis V: Global assessment of functioning (the GAF scale)

DSM-IV has as its fifth axis a 0–100 scale rating psychological, social and occupational functioning. Detailed descriptions for each centile band are given by DSM-IV; for a useful summary, see LaBruzza and Mendez-Villarrubia (1994). Such a scale may be particularly useful in tracking and evaluating treatment and progress in treatment. In outline, the bands are:

- 91–100 – superior functioning;
- 81–90 – good functioning in all areas; minimal problems or symptoms;
- 71–80 – transient symptoms or mild impairment in relation to stressors;
- 61–70 – mild symptoms *or* some difficulty in functioning; child may occasionally steal or truant;
- 51–60 – moderate symptoms *or* moderate difficulty in functioning, e.g. child with few friends, some symptoms of depression;
- 41–50 – serious symptoms, e.g. suicidal ideation, frequent stealing, incapacitating anxiety, severe obsessional rituals, *or* any serious impairment in functioning – e.g. difficulty attending school, no friends;
- 31–40 – impaired reality testing or communication, *or* major impairment in several areas, e.g. no friends, school failure or non-attendance, out of control at home, beats up younger children;
- 21–30 – behaviour considerably influenced by delusions or hallucinations *or* serious impairment in communication or judgement *or* inability to function in almost all areas;
- 11–20 – some danger of hurting self or others, *or* occasionally fails to maintain minimal personal hygiene (e.g. smearing faeces), *or* gross impairment of communication;
- 1–10 – persistent danger of severely hurting self or others *or* persistent inability to maintain minimal personal hygiene *or* serious suicidal act with clear expectation of death.

Towards a formulation

The clinician should by this time have sufficient information with which to draft a provisional cognitive behavioural formulation. However, such a formulation also needs to take into account the family-systemic aspects of the problem.

The basic five-component cognitive behavioural model

Using Padesky's basic five-component cognitive behavioural model (see Figure 4.1), the clinician can then annotate the model with the presenting symptoms. According to the age and understanding of the child, this exercise might be carried out in discussion with the child and their family (see Figure 4.2).

The advantage of this exercise is that it establishes from the start a collaborative relationship between the therapist, the young person and the family, and helps them see the link between thoughts, emotions, behaviour and somatic symptoms.

An extended model

An extended model (see Figure 4.3) allows the clinician to elaborate on the formulation. This model, although more complex, could also be annotated as a collaborative exercise with the family. For example, for our hypothetical school-refuser, we might begin to annotate Figure 4.3 as follows.

Acquisition of fear or anxiety

- *Modelling* – father models avoidant behaviour.
- *Direct conditioning* – severe bullying at school.
- *Instruction/information* – parent covertly conveys to the child that the child is vulnerable, lacks coping skills.

Beliefs

- *The child's core beliefs* – 'The world is threatening'; 'I am vulnerable'; 'I won't be able to cope.'

Avoidance

- *Behavioural avoidance* – child shrinks from attempting to return to school.

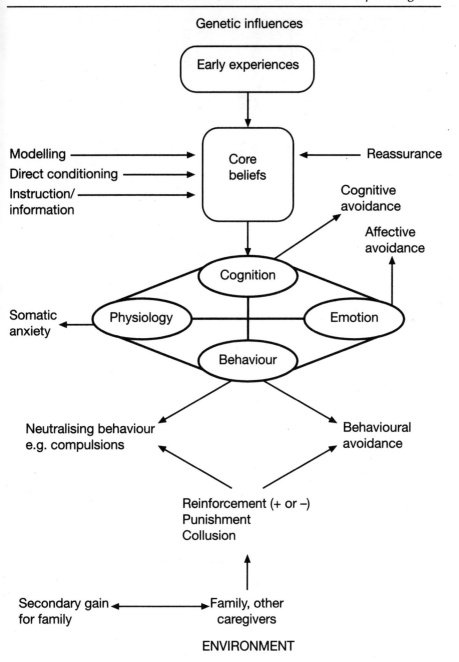

Figure 4.3 **Anxiety disorders: Predisposition, acquisition and maintenance–elaboration of Padesky's five-component model**

	Acquisition	Maintenance	Resolution
The Child	Predisposing vulnerability ? genetic influences	Behavioural avoidance Core beliefs concerning threat, personal vulnerability Cognitive distortions, e.g. catastrophising	Child has good rapport with the therapist Child prepared to attempt to confront difficult situations Child amenable to cognitive restructuring
The Family	Father suffers from an anxiety disorder – models avoidant behaviour	Parental anxiety about the child and child's ability to cope in school Belief that the child is 'ill', vulnerable	Family engaged Motivated to attend sessions and resolve problems No serious family psychopathology Parents motivated to support each other
Extra-familial Environment	Severe bullying by a clique of fellow pupils at school	Bullying continues Child isolated from friends in neighbourhood following recent house move	School maintains good liaison with family and with therapist Headteacher enthusiastic and mobilises school's pastoral resources

Figure 4.4 A hypothetical case of school refusal: Application of a matrix model

- *Cognitive avoidance* – child does not want to think or talk about school.
- *Reassurance* – child frequently asks for reassurance, mother responds by giving reassurance.

Contingencies

- *Behavioural reinforcement* – positive reinforcement (cuddle) from parent when child runs back home from school.

Acquisition, maintenance and resolution: A matrix model

In order to plan treatment effectively, it is important that the therapist looks at the factors which could be operable in the resolution of the problem, as well as its acquisition and maintenance. A matrix model (see Figure 4.4) considers the factors in the child, his family, and the wider environment in the acquisition, maintenance and resolution of the problem.

Conclusion

The assessment and treatment of anxiety disorder is a rapidly-developing field, and all theories and treatment modalities are in the process of modification in the light of experience and research data. Anxiety manifests itself in various ways (physiological, cognitive, emotional and behavioural) and often varies markedly across situations and according to context. Furthermore, the therapist needs to consider the family-systemic aspects of anxiety disorders in order to maximise understanding and to construct the most comprehensive formulation. It is necessary, therefore, to glean information from as many sources as possible.

References

Achenbach, T.M. & Edelbrock, C.S. (1983) *Manual for the Child Behaviour Checklist and Revised Child Behaviour Profile*, Burlington, VT: Department of Psychiatry, University of Vermont.

Achenbach, T.M., McConaughy, S.H. & Howell, C.T. (1987) 'Child and adolescent behavioural and emotional problems: Implications of cross-informant correlations for situational specificity', *Psychological Bulletin*, 101, pp.213–32.

American Psychiatric Association (1994) *Diagnostic and Statistical Manual of Mental Disorders: Fourth Edition (DSM-IV)*, Washington, DC: American Psychiatric Association.

Bandura, A. (1969) *Principles of Behaviour Modification*, New York: Holt, Rinehart and Winston.

Barrios, B.A. & Hartmann, D.P. (1988) 'Fears and anxieties', in Mash, E.J. & Terdal, L.G. (eds) *Behavioural Assessment of Childhood Disorders*, New York: Guilford Press, pp.196–264.

Barrios, B.A., Hartmann, D.P. & Shigetomi, C. (1981) 'Fears and anxieties in children', in Mash, E.J. & Terdal, L.G. (eds) *Behavioural Assessment of Childhood Disorders* (1st edn), New York: Guilford Press, pp.259–304.

Beck, A.T., Ward, C.H., Mendelson, M., Mock, J. & Erbaugh, J. (1961) 'An inventory for measuring depression', *Archives of General Psychiatry*, 4, pp.561–71.

Bernstein, G.A. & Borchardt, C.M. (1990) 'Anxiety disorders', in Garfinkel, B.D., Carlson, G.A. & Weller, E.B. (eds) *Psychiatric Disorder in Children and Adolescents*, Orlando, FL: W.B. Saunders, pp.64–83.

Bernstein, G.A. & Borchardt, C.M. (1991) 'Anxiety disorders of childhood and adolescence: A critical review', *Journal of the American Academy of Child and Adolescent Psychiatry*, 30(4), pp.519–32.

Bernstein, G.A. & Garfinkel, B.D. (1986) 'School phobia: The overlap of affective and anxiety disorders', *Journal of the American Academy of Child and Adolescent Psychiatry*, 25(2), pp.235–41.

Bernstein, G.A. & Garfinkel, B.D. (1988) 'Pedigrees, functioning, and psychopathology in families of school phobic children', *American Journal of Psychiatry*, 145, pp.70–4.

Bernstein, G.A., Garfinkel, B.D. & Hoberman, H. (1989) 'Self-reported anxiety in adolescents', *American Journal of Psychiatry*, 146, pp.384–6.

Bernstein, G.A., Svingen, P.H. & Garfinkel, B.D. (1990) 'School phobia: Patterns of family functioning', *Journal of the American Academy of Child and Adolescent Psychiatry*, 29(1), pp.24–30.   •

Bierman, K.L. (1984) 'Cognitive development and clinical interviews with children', in Lahey, B.B. & Kazdin, A.E. (eds) *Advances in Clinical Child Psychology*, Vol.6, New York: Plenum Press, pp.217–50.

Clark, D.B., Smith, M.G., Neighbors, B.D., Skerlec, L.M. & Randall, J. (1994) 'Anxiety disorders in adolescents: Characteristics, prevalence, comorbidities', *Clinical Psychology Review*, 14(2), pp.113–38.

Clark, D.M. (1989) 'Anxiety states: Panic and generalised anxiety', in Hawton, K., Salkovskis, P.M., Kirk, J. & Clark., D.M. (eds) *Cognitive Behaviour Therapy for Psychiatric Problems*, Oxford: Oxford University Press.

Connors, C.K. (1994) 'Connors Rating Scales', in Maruish, M.E. (ed.) *The Use of Psychological Testing for Treatment Planning and Outcome Measurement*, Hillsdale, N.J.: Lawrence Erlbaum.

Costello, A.J., Edelbrock, C.S., Kalas, R., Dulcan, M.K. & Claris, S.H. (1984) 'Development and testing of the NIMH diagnostic interview for children (DISC) in a clinic population: Final report', Rockville, M.D.: Center for Epidemiological Studies, NIMH.

Degonda, M. & Angst, J. (1993) 'The Zurich Study XX: Social phobia and agoraphobia', *European Archives of Psychiatry and Clinical Neuroscience*, 243(2), pp.95–102.

Deltito, J.A. & Hahn, R. (1993) 'A three-generational presentation of separation anxiety in childhood with agoraphobia in adulthood', *Psychopharmacology Bulletin*, 29(2), pp.189–93.

Dumas, J.E. & LaFreniere, P.J. (1993) 'Mother–child relationships as sources of support or stress: A comparison of competent, average, aggressive and anxious dyads', *Child Development*, 64(6), pp.1,732–54.

Edelbrock, C., Costello, A.J., Duncan, M.K. & Kalas, R. (1985) 'Age differences in the reliability of the psychiatric interview of the child', *Child Development*, 56, pp.265–75.

Eminson, M. (1993) 'Assessment in child and adolescent psychiatry', in Black, D. & Cottrell, D. (eds) *Seminars in Child & Adolescent Psychiatry*, Royal College of Psychiatrists.

Finch, A.J., Saylor, C.F. & Edwards, G.L. (1985) 'Children's Depression Inventory: Sex and grade norms for normal children', *Journal of Consulting and Clinical Psychology*, 53, pp.424–5.

Francis, G., Last, C.G. & Strauss, C.C. (1992) 'Avoidant disorder and social phobia in children and adolescents', *Journal of the American Academy of Child and Adolescent Psychiatry*, 31(6), pp.1,086–9.

Fyer, A.J. (1993) 'Heritability of social anxiety: A brief review', *Clinical Psychiatry*, 54(Supplement), pp.10–12.

Graham, P. (1991) *Child Psychiatry: A Developmental Approach* (2nd edn), Oxford: Oxford Medical Publications, pp.166–79.

Harter, S. (1985) *Manual for the Self-Perception Profile for Children*, Denver: University of Denver.

Harter, S. (1988) *Manual for the Self-Perception Profile for Adolescents*, Denver: University of Denver.

Harter, S. & Nowakowski, M. (1987) *Manual for the Dimensions of Depression Profile for Children and Adolescents*, Denver: University of Denver.

Herjanic, B. & Reich, W. (1982) 'Development of a structured psychiatric interview for children: Agreement between child and parent on individual symptoms', *Journal of Abnormal Child Psychology*, 10, pp.307–24.

Horowitz, M.J. (1976) *Stress Response Syndromes*, New York: Jason Aronson.

Horowitz, M.J., Wilner, N. & Alvarez, W. (1979) 'Impact of Event Scale: A measure of subjective distress', *Psychosomatic Medicine*, 41, pp.209–18.

Kazdin, A.E. (1986) 'Research designs and methodology', in Garfield, S.L. & Bergin, A.E. (eds) *Handbook of Psychotherapy and Behaviour Change*, New York: John Wiley, pp.23–9.

Kazdin, A.E., French, N.H., Unis, A.S., Esveldt-Dawson, K. & Sherick, R.B. (1983) 'Hopelessness, depression, and suicidal intent among psychiatrically disturbed in-patient children', *Journal of Consulting and Clinical Psychology*, 51, pp.501–10.

Kendall, P.C. (1994) 'Treating anxiety disorders in children: Results of a randomised clinical trial', *Journal of Consulting and Clinical Psychology*, 62(1), pp.100–10.

Kendall, P.C. & Brady, E.U. (1995) 'Comorbidity in the anxiety disorders of childhood: Implications for validity and clinical significance', in Craig, K.D. & Dobson, K.S. (eds) *Anxiety and Depression in Adults and Children*, Banff International Behavioural Science Series, Thousand Oaks, CA: Sage Publications.

Kendall, P.C. & Ronan, K.R. (1990a) 'Assessment of children's anxieties, fears and phobias: Cognitive-behavioural models and methods', in Reynolds, C.R. & Camphaus, R.W. (eds) *Handbook of Psychological and Educational Assessment of Children: Personality, Behaviour and Context*, New York: Guilford Press.

Kendall, P.C. & Ronan, K.R. (1990b) *Children's Anxious Self Statement Questionnaire (CASSQ)*, Philadelphia, PA: Department of Psychology, Temple University.

Kendall, P.C., Cantwell, D. & Kasdin, A.E. (1989) 'Depression in children and adolescents: Assessment issues and recommendations', *Cognitive Therapy and Research*, 13, pp.109–46.

Kendall, P.C., Pellegrini, D.S. & Urbain, E.S. (1981) 'Approaches to assessment for cognitive-behavioural interventions in children', in Kendall, P.C. & Hollon, S.D. (eds) *Assessment Strategies for Cognitive Behavioural Interventions*, London: Academic Press, pp.227–85.

Kendall, P.C., Chansky, T.E., Friedman, M., Kim, R., Kortlander, E., Sessa, F.M. & Siqueland, L. (1991) 'Treating anxiety disorders in children and adolescents', in Kendall, P.C. (ed.) *Child and Adolescent Therapy: Cognitive-Behavioural Procedures*, New York: Guilford Press.

Kendall, P.C., Chansky, T.E., Kane, M., Kim, R., Kortlander, E., Ronan, K., Sessa, F. & Siqueland, L. (1992) *Anxiety Disorders in Youth: Cognitive Behavioural Interventions*, Needham Heights, MA: Allyn & Bacon.

Kessler, R.C., McGonagle, K.A., Zhao, S., Nelson, C.B., Hughes, M., Eshleman, S., Wittchen, H.U. & Kendler, K.S. (1994) 'Lifetime and 12 month prevalence of DSM-III-R psychiatric disorders in the United States: Results from the National Comorbidity Study', *Archives of General Psychiatry*, 51(1), pp.8–19.

King, N.J., Gullone, E. & Ollendick, T.H. (1991) 'Manifest anxiety and fearfulness in children and adolescents', *Journal of Genetic Psychology*, 153(1), pp.63–73.

King, N.J., Hamilton, D.I. & Ollendick, T.H. (1988) *Children's Phobias: A Behavioural Perspective*, Chichester: John Wiley.

Kirk, J. (1989) 'Cognitive-behavioural assessment', in Hawton, K., Salkovskis, P.M., Kirk, J. & Clark, D.M. (eds) *Cognitive Behaviour Therapy for Psychiatric Problems*, Oxford: Oxford University Press.

Kovacs, M. (1981) 'Rating Scales to assess depression in school aged children', *Acta Paedopsychiatrica*, 46, pp.305–15.

Kuehlwein, K.T. & Rosen, H. (eds) (1993) *Cognitive Therapies in Action: Evolving Clinical Practice*, San Franscisco: Jossey-Bass.

LaBruzza, A.L. & Mendez-Villarrubia, J.M. (1994) *Using DSM-IV: A Clinician's Guide to Psychiatric Diagnosis*, Northvale, NJ: Jason Aronson.

March, J., Parker, J. & Connors, C. (forthcoming a) 'The Multidimensional Anxiety Scale for Children (MASC): Reliability and validity', unpublished manuscript.

March, J., Stallings, P., Parker, J., Terry, R. & Connors, C. (forthcoming b) 'The Multidimensional Anxiety Scale for Children (MASC): Development and factor structure', unpublished manuscript.

Murphy, G.C., Hudson, A.M., King, N.J. & Remenyi, A. (1985) 'An interview schedule for use in the behavioural assessment of children's problems', *Behaviour Change*, 2, pp.6–12.

Neeman, J. & Harter, S. (1986) *Manual for the Self Perception Profile for College Students*, Denver: University of Denver.

Ollendick, T.H. (1983) 'Reliability and validity of the revised fear survey schedule for children (FSSC-R)', *Behaviour Research and Therapy*, 21, pp.685–92.

Ollendick, T.H. (1995) 'Assessment of anxiety and phobic disorders in children', in Craig, K.D. & Dobson, K.S. (eds) *Anxiety and Depression in Adults and Children*, Banff International Behavioural Science Series, Thousand Oaks, CA: Sage Publications.

Ollendick, T.H. & King, N.J. (1991) 'Origins of childhood fears: An evaluation of Rachman's theory of fear acquisition', *Behaviour Research and Therapy*, 29(2), pp.117–23.

Ollendick, T.H. & King, N.J. (1994) 'Fears and their levels of interference in adolescents', *Behaviour Research and Therapy*, 32(6), pp.635–8.

Ollendick, T.H., King, N.J. & Frary, R.B. (1989) 'Fears in children and adolescents: Reliability and generalisability across gender, age and nationality', *Behaviour Research and Therapy*, 27(1), pp.19–26.

Padesky, C.A. & Mooney, K.A. (1986) 'Clinical tip: Presenting the cognitive model to clients', *International Cognitive Therapy Newsletter*, 6, pp.13–14.

Parker, J., March, J. & Connors, C. (forthcoming) 'The Multidimensional Anxiety Scale for Children (MASC): Confirmatory factor analysis', unpublished manuscript.

Persons, J.B. (1989) *Cognitive Therapy in Practice: A Case Formulation Approach*, New York: W.W. Norton.

Pynoos, R.S. (1990) 'Post-traumatic stress disorder in children and adolescents', in Garfinkel, B.D., Carlson, G.A. & Weller, E.B. (eds) *Psychiatric Disorder in Children and Adolescents*, Orlando, FL: W.B. Saunders, pp.48–63.

Pynoos, R.S., Frederick, C., Nader, K., Arroyo, W., Steinberg, A., Eth, S., Nunez, F. & Fairbanks, L. (1987) 'Life threat and post-traumatic stress in school-age children', *Archives of General Psychiatry*, 44, pp.1,057–63.

Rachman, S. (1977) 'The conditioning theory of fear acquisition: A critical examination', *Behaviour Research and Therapy*, 15, pp.375–87.

Reinherz, H.Z., Giaconia, R.M., Lefkowitz, E.S., Pakiz, B. & Frost, A.K. (1993) 'Prevalence of psychiatric disorders in a community population of older adolescents', *Journal of the American Academy of Child and Adolescent Psychiatry*, 32(2), pp.369–77.

Reynolds, C.R. & Richmond, B.O. (1978) ' "What I think and feel": A revised measure of children's manifest anxiety', *Journal of Abnormal Child Psychology*, 6(2), pp.271–80.

Ronan, K.R., Kendall, P.C. & Rowe, M. (1994) 'Negative affectivity in children: Development and validation of a self-statement questionnaire', *Cognitive Therapy and Research*, 18(6).

Salkovskis, P.M. & Kirk, J. (1989) 'Obsessional disorders', in Hawton, K., Salkovskis, P.M. & Clark, D.M. (eds) *Cognitive Behaviour Therapy for Psychiatric Problems*, Oxford: Oxford University Press.

Saylor, C.F., Finch, A., Spirito, A. & Bennett, B. (1984) 'The Children's Depression Inventory: A systematic examination of psychometric properties', *Journal of Consulting and Clinical Psychology*, 52, pp.955–67.

Schwartz, E. & Perry, B.D. (1994) 'The post traumatic response in children and adolescents', *Psychiatric Clinics of North America*, 17(2), pp.311–26.

Scott, M.J. & Stradling, S.G. (1992) *Counselling for Post-Traumatic Stress Disorder*, London: Sage Publications.

Silverman, W. (1987) *Anxiety Disorder Interview Schedule for Children (ADIS)*, Albany, NY: Graywind Publications.

Silverman, W. & Albano, A.M. (in press) *Anxiety Disorders Interview Schedule for Parent and Child*, San Antonio, TX: Graywind Publications.

Silverman, W. & Kearney, C.A. (1992) 'Listening to our clinical partners: Informing researchers about children's fears and phobias', *Journal of Behavioural Therapy and Experimental Psychiatry*, 23(2), pp.71–6.

Spielberger, C.D., Gorsuch, R.L. & Lushene, R.E. (1970) *Manual for the State-Trait Anxiety Inventory*, Palo Alto, CA: Consulting Psychologists Press.

Stallings, P. & March, J.S. (1995) 'Assessment', in March, J.S. (ed.) *Anxiety Disorders in Children and Adolescents*, New York: Guilford Press, pp.125–47.

Walk, R.D. (1956) 'Self-ratings of fear in a fear-involving situation', *Journal of Abnormal and Social Psychology*, 52, pp.171–9.

Walker, E.A., Katon, W.J., Hansom, J., Harrop-Griffiths, J., Holm, L., Jones, M.L., Hickok, L. & Jemelka, R.P. (1992) 'Medical and psychiatric symptoms in women with childhood sexual abuse', *Psychosomatic Medicine*, 54(6), pp.658–64.

Werry, J.S. (1986) 'Diagnosis and assessment', in Gittelman, R. (ed.) *Anxiety Disorders in Childhood*, New York: Guilford Press, pp.73–100.

World Health Organisation (1992) *The ICD-10 Classification of Mental and Behavioural Disorders*, Geneva: World Health Organisation.

Yule, W. & Udwin, O. (1991) 'Screening child survivors for post-traumatic stress disorders: Experiences from the "Jupiter" sinking', *British Journal of Clinical Psychology*, 30, pp.131–8.

5 Assessing and monitoring anxiety in children

David Jones

Anxiety is a central construct, both in theories of personality and in psychiatric classification systems of disorders of childhood. The range of different tests and questionnaires which have been devised to measure anxiety levels in children bears testimony to the multifaceted nature of the construct. One of the most important distinctions is that between state-anxiety and trait-anxiety (Cattell & Scheier, 1961; Spielberger, 1966). State-anxiety refers to a transitory reaction to stress characterised by unpleasant subjective feelings of tension and apprehension. Objective measurement also confirms associated changes in autonomic nervous system activity. Trait-anxiety refers to the more stable characteristic of degree of anxiety-proneness. The two are highly correlated, since children with high levels of trait-anxiety are likely to experience state-anxiety more frequently and in a wider range of situations than other children.

Adopting a combined ethological and developmental viewpoint of anxiety and fear, it can be seen that they have an adaptive function in the early years of life, inhibiting dangerous exploration and unnecessary contact with potentially harmful strangers. As childhood progresses, appropriate anxiety levels appear to play a part in facilitating the development of socialisation and the acquisition of moral codes. In different ways, anxiety is also likely to be involved in the need for affiliation with others, the need for achievement and the attainment of culturally-acceptable competitiveness.

On the negative side, it is clear that high levels of anxiety inhibit exploration and social development in infants and pre-school children. Effects on social functioning and problems relating to difficulty in separation from parental figures may be even more noticeable in older children. In some cases, specific phobias and avoidance behaviour directly attributable to anxieties may prevent school attendance or inhibit learning. The relations between anxiety levels and academic attainments in school-age children are generally complex, and will be discussed in more detail later. Persistent high levels of anxiety on the majority of days over a period of six months or more are referred to as 'overanxious disorder of childhood' in the recent DSM-IV classification of disorders (American Psychiatric Association, 1994). The major factors of the disturbance vary in different children, but include restlessness or feeling on edge, being easily fatigued, concentration difficulty, irritability, muscle tension and sleep disturbance.

A psychometric perspective on the structure of personality allows anxiety to be seen in the context of other measurable dimensions. For many years, the choice of model was between a multi-trait interpretation of personality such as that suggested by Cattell (1973) and the two-factor model proposed by Eysenck (1970). Cattell's 16PF identifies 15 traits and intelligence. Several of the source traits appear to measure aspects of anxiety, and higher-order factoring produces a major anxiety factor along with a factor reflecting sociability. In the Eysenck model, anxiety is a major component of the normal–neuroticism dimension, the other dimension being extroversion–introversion. Eysenck and Eysenck (1975) added the P-Scale, or 'toughmindedness', as a third dimension of personality.

Recent practical and theoretical developments suggest that personality should be construed in terms of five broad factors which have quickly come to be known as the 'Big Five' (Digman, 1990; Goldberg, 1993; Hampson, 1995). The factors are:

1   *extroversion* (or surgency), which identifies traits such as extroverted–introverted, talkative–quiet and bold–timid;
2   *agreeableness*, which is based on characteristics such as agreeable–disagreeable, kind–unkind and selfish–unselfish;
3   *conscientiousness*, reflecting traits such as organised–disorganised, hardworking–lazy, reliable–unreliable, thorough–careless and practical–impractical;
4   *neuroticism* (or emotional stability), based on traits such as stable–unstable, relaxed–tense, calm–angry and unemotional–emotional;
5   *openness to experience* (or culture, or intellect), which reflects cognitive ability, level of sophistication, creativity, curiosity and position on an analytical–unanalytical cognitive style.

There is as yet relatively little systematic work on the measurement of some of these factors in children, so it remains to be seen whether the full model will be useful. Intuitively, it would seem important also to know the extent to which a child identified as anxious is also agreeable, conscientious and introverted, and to what extent these other characteristics remain stable over time.

Methods of measurement

Measures of anxiety, like all other psychometric measures, should meet the criteria of having satisfactory levels of reliability and validity. Reliability, in the sense of stability of the measure over time, is an essential prerequisite of trait measures. Assessing the reliability of tests of state-anxiety depends more on demonstrating consistency across similar situations. Validity is essentially the extent to which a measure reflects the construct identified by the test designer.

It is possible to classify measures of anxiety in children into at least seven groups.

The largest group consists of questionnaires or inventories requiring direct responses by the children. Questionnaires are used to measure and monitor trait-anxiety, state-anxiety and specific anxieties and fears as symptoms of clinical disorders.

A second group of measures consists of rating scales of children's behaviour to be completed by parents, teachers and other adults who have had opportunities to observe the children. Such rating scales are particularly useful when the requirement is to monitor change during or following therapeutic intervention.

A third group includes projective tests which involve interpretation of children's responses to standard test material or a set of instructions. Usually, the administrators of projective tests need to be trained in the method and committed to a psychodynamic model of development.

A fourth approach is to use objective tests which are not in themselves direct measures of anxiety, but which may allow inferences on anxiety level to be made from an analysis of test performance.

A fifth group consists of physiological techniques for measuring arousal and autonomic nervous system activity.

In the sixth group, we will consider estimation of anxiety from sociometric measures of children's popularity or loneliness within their peer groups.

Finally, there is a small but important group of measures of attachment, security and anxiety in social relationships between children of different ages and their primary caregivers.

Questionnaire methods

The majority of questionnaires used to assess anxiety in children have been derived from similar instruments developed earlier to assess anxiety in adults. Such an approach does not guarantee that the same construct is being measured in children and adults. Anxiety questionnaires tend to consist of a series of items which describe how the child feels about themself, about interactions with others or about being in specific situations. Sometimes, there is an attempt to control for response bias in agreeing or disagreeing with statements by a careful balancing of the wording of the items.

Many anxiety questionnaires include a 'lie scale', consisting of items designed to detect when a child is attempting to fake responses to present themself in a good light. There is a problem in the interpretation of high lie scale scores obtained by children, since they sometimes reflect social immaturity rather than an intention to deceive. A consequence is that scores on anxiety and other personality dimensions must be viewed with caution when children's lie scale scores are one standard deviation or more above the mean for the age group.

The Revised Children's Manifest Anxiety Scale (RCMAS)

The RCMAS (Reynolds & Richmond, 1978; Reynolds & Paget, 1981) is one of the more widely-used questionnaires in clinical research studies. It is a revision of the Children's Manifest Anxiety Scale (CMAS – Castaneda et al., 1956), which is derived from the Manifest Anxiety Scale (MAS – Taylor, 1953). The theoretical background is of interest, since the MAS itself was based on items selected from the Minnesota Multiphasic Personality Inventory (MMPI).

The RCMAS, in common with the CMAS, is a measure of general anxiety, and should be regarded as a trait measure. It does not identify the specific situations in which children experience anxiety. Examples of items in the RCMAS are: 'I worry about what my parents will say to me' and 'I worry about what other people think about me.' In all, the scale contains 37 items, including a short lie scale.

The General Anxiety Scale for Children (GASC)

The GASC (Sarason et al., 1960) is another well-established measure of trait-anxiety. Examples of items are: 'If you were to climb a ladder, would you worry about falling off it?' and 'Do you think you worry more than other boys and girls?' The GASC has been used in conjunction with the Test Anxiety Scale for Children, which will be discussed later in this section.

The Eysenck scales

The Junior Eysenck Personality Inventory (JEPI – S.B.G. Eysenck, 1965) is the children's version of the Eysenck Personality Inventory (EPI), which measures the two major personality dimensions, neuroticism (or emotionality) and extroversion–introversion. The questionnaire is intended for use with children in the age range 7–16 years and has separate norms for boys and girls. The neuroticism scale is essentially a measure of trait or general anxiety. The junior version of the Eysenck Personality Questionnaire (EPQ – Eysenck & Eysenck, 1975) is similar to the JEPI but also provides a measure of 'toughmindedness' (the P-scale). Norms are available for the age range 7–15 years. On both questionnaires, the means suggest an increase in anxiety with age for girls, but little change for boys.

The IPAT scales

The pioneering work on assessment by Cattell and his associates at the Institute for Personality and Ability Testing (IPAT) in Illinois has resulted in a series of multi-trait measures, of which the best-known is the 16PF for adults. The Children's Personality Questionnaire (CPQ – Porter & Cattell, 1963) measures 14 source traits, including intelligence, for children aged 8–12 years. It is possible to calculate scores for higher-order factors of anxiety and extroversion. Two forms of the test are available, and administration of both forms is recommended for clinical use. However, each form can take up to 50 minutes to complete. Questions in the CPQ are in a forced-choice form, for example 'Do you have many friends or just a few good friends?' Cattell considers that the test estimates level of free-floating, manifest anxiety, which may be influenced by long-term and situational variables.

Children in the age range 6–8 years are covered by the Early School Personality Questionnaire (ESPQ – Coan & Cattell, 1966). In this version, the items are read aloud to the children, who enter their responses on record forms which are well-designed and easy to use. Gillis (1980) has devised the Child Anxiety Scale, based on the criterion of the ESPQ second-order anxiety factor. The test has 20 items which are read out to individuals or small groups of children. Each item is clearly identified on the record form by a drawing, for example of a butterfly or a spoon, to minimise the chance of mistakes in entering the responses. This is a useful, quick screening test for anxiety level for children in the age range 5–12 years.

The State-Trait Anxiety Inventory for Children (STAIC)

The STAIC (Spielberger et al., 1970b) consists of two separate self-report scales, one to measure state-anxiety (A-State) and one to measure trait-anxiety (A-Trait). The A-State scale investigates how children are feeling at the time they are actually taking the test. There are 20 items, and for each statement the child is required to choose from three boxes, for example 'I feel ... "very frightened", "frightened" or "not frightened".' For half of the items, the 'very' box indicates the presence of anxiety, and for other items it indicates the absence of anxiety, as in 'I feel ... "very satisfied".' The A-Trait scale has 20 statements requiring responses in terms of how the child generally feels: for example for the statement 'I feel unhappy' there is a choice from 'hardly ever', 'sometimes' or 'often'. The STAIC is intended for children aged 9–12 years. Adolescents can be given the State-Trait Anxiety Inventory (STAI), which is the adult version (Spielberger et al., 1970a).

Measures of test anxiety

The more situationally-specific concept of anxiety experienced in the classroom environment or in test-taking situations has given rise to several tests. The Test Anxiety Scale for Children (TASC – Sarason et al., 1960) consists of 30 items, for example 'When the teacher says that she is going to find out how much you have learned, does your heart beat faster?' Children who respond positively to 10 to 15 items are considered moderately test-anxious, and those who score more than 15 are classified as highly test-anxious.

The School Anxiety Scale (SAS – Phillips, 1978) includes many of the TASC items, but is a longer test, having 74 items in all. Both the TASC and the SAS appear to have similar multifactorial structures, providing possible measures of fear of assertiveness and self-expression, test anxiety, lack of confidence in meeting expectations of others and physiological reactivity to low levels of stress. It can be useful to attempt to monitor these components separately in children who appear to be incapacitated by anxiety in the school situation.

Numerous studies have reported a negative correlation between test anxiety scores and academic achievement (Sarason, 1980). The pattern of emphasis placed on different subjects at school may affect the relation between anxiety and attainment: for example some studies report a negative correlation between TASC scores and attainment in arithmetic, but not in reading. The effects of high test anxiety seem more likely to be debilitating when the child perceives the situation as threatening or evaluative. There is some evidence that moderate levels of anxiety may facilitate rather than impair overall performance in intellectually able children and adolescents.

Behavioural rating scales

The clinician will always need to exercise judgement in interpreting scores obtained from rating scales completed by parents. The Child Behavior Checklist (CBCL – Achenbach & Edelbrock, 1983) has been widely used and has good test-retest reliability. In all, there are 113 items, including three scales providing measures of social competence in activities, social behaviour and school behaviour. The main section provides scores on nine scales dealing with specific categories, of which somatic complaints and social withdrawal are perhaps the most relevant for the assessment of behaviours related to anxiety. Two higher-order factor scales provide information on internalising and externalising.

A shorter multidimensional rating scale for completion by parents is the Connors Parent Symptom Questionnaire (PSQ – Goyette et al., 1978). The 48-item version of the PSQ includes a short anxiety scale and a measure of psychosomatic problems, as well as hyperactivity–impulsivity and conduct problems. A brief rating scale covering aspects of health and behaviour for school-age children has been standardised by Rutter et al. (1970) to identify behaviour problems and emotional difficulties. For younger children, a suitable rating scale for completion by parents is the Preschool Behaviour Checklist (McGuire & Richman, 1988).

There are also several rating scales for completion by teachers which provide measures of children's anxiety levels. The Connors Teacher Rating Scale (TRS – Goyette et al., 1978) has been widely used to help identify children with hyperactivity, although some of the items focus on anxiety. Similarly, the Rutter (B2) Rating Scale for Teachers is an easily-completed screening measure of a range of difficulties experienced by children, including anxiety (Rutter et al., 1970).

The Bristol Social Adjustment Guides (BSAG – Stott, 1974) have been used widely as a checklist to be completed by teachers, mainly to provide an index of maladjustment in the school setting. Stott suggests that a measure of school situation anxiety can be obtained from ratings of both overreacting and underreacting behaviours.

Projective tests

Psycho-analytic theories of projection focus on the need to understand unconscious processes before it is possible to explain disturbed behaviour. It is claimed that projective tests provide a means for sampling underlying processes and emotions, even though interpretation of responses has to take account of the child's intelligence and awareness of external reality. Many psychologists are dismissive of projective tests on the grounds that it is almost impossible to establish their validity. There is also the problem that projective techniques are often quite lengthy procedures, and interpretation requires special training and acceptance of a psychodynamic model. There is evidence that children with problems in clinic populations sometimes perform differently from other children on projective tests, and also that such tests can be useful for screening suspected victims of sexual abuse.

The Children's Apperception Test (CAT – Bellak & Bellak, 1957) has been widely used with school-age children. The child is shown a series of cards, and for each one is asked to describe the events leading up to the picture, what is happening at the present, and what is likely to happen. Interpretation of anxieties includes attention to perceived threat in the stories, as well as comments about potential loss. The CAT is a children's version of the Thematic Apperception Test (TAT – Bellak and Bellak, 1957), which is still sometimes used with adolescents.

No discussion of projective tests would be complete without some mention of the Rorschach ink blot test (Francis-Williams, 1968). The test cards deliberately lack obvious meaning, although there is symmetry and a variation in complexity, shading and the use of colour. Interpretation of children's responses is a complex task, which includes an attempt to assess cognitive functioning as well as anxieties and fears. Critics argue that the same information could be obtained more quickly in a carefully-structured clinical interview.

The Object Relations Technique (ORT – Phillipson, 1973) has become more popular than the TAT for use with the adolescent age group, partly because the stimulus material is more age-appropriate. The ORT again involves a storytelling procedure in response to 13 cards arranged in three series, each depicting a scene involving one person, two people, three people and a group. There is a progression of detail across the series, from soft tones and hazy figures to stronger contrasts, and finally the use of colour and more realism.

When children are reluctant to communicate verbally, it is possible to make interpretations about emotional difficulties by analysis of their drawings (Cummings, 1986). Children are usually prepared to draw people they are concerned about, but as with projective testing generally, the validity of interpretations remains open to criticism. One approach involves a detailed analysis of three groups of features in the drawings. These are quality signs, which include overall size of the figures, special features such as position and size of arms, legs and other body parts, and omissions of specific body parts (Koppitz, 1968). Analysis of young children's drawings of their families can provide insight into aspects of anxiety around sibling rivalry and the relative importance of other family members to the child. Cautious interpretation of children's drawings can sometimes provide additional information when there are suspicions of sexual abuse.

It is debatable whether interpretation of structured doll and toy play situations should be labelled as a psychometric procedure. Such an approach does come under the heading of 'projective techniques', and there is an extensive literature on the subject (Greenspan, 1981). Highly-specialised techniques have been developed using anatomically complete dolls to explore the possibility of sexual abuse in young or non-communicative children (Vizard & Tranter, 1988).

Objective techniques

This category is somewhat open-ended. It includes an evaluation of performance on a range of tests of speed, motor skill and decision-taking which are not in themselves direct measures of anxiety. Even such tasks as doing mental arithmetic problems, solving anagrams and paired-associated learning for word lists of different difficulty levels may be included. The general assumption is that anxious children are more likely to show fluctuations in their performance levels than other children. It is also hypothesised that, in general, anxious children will do well on relatively easy tasks, but that their performance breaks down as task complexity increases. The validity of inferences about anxiety level based on such observations of performance is questionable. There is little in the way of normative data on the topic. A similar criticism applies to inferences about anxiety levels based on interpretation of the pattern of scores obtained from a battery of cognitive tests. Low scores on tests involving concentration or speed relative to other measures may indicate state-anxiety, but other explanations for such discrepancies should also be considered.

Physiological techniques

An evaluation of the psychophysiology of anxiety is beyond the scope of this chapter. Unfortunately, distinctions between arousal level and emotionality are sometimes not clear in the literature, and care must be taken when comparisons are made between changes in physiological activity in highly-anxious children and those in control samples. Almost certainly, anxiety involves the limbic system and the reticular activating system in a complex interaction with both the sympathetic and para-sympathetic branches of the autonomic nervous system. Individual differences in reactivity to stressful stimuli and response specificity are at least partly explained by the additional involvement of cortical activity, reflecting conditioning and past emotional experiences.

Physical symptoms are readily detectable when a child has an acute anxiety attack, and it scarcely needs complex equipment to monitor rapid breathing, tremor, perspiration, dizziness, vomiting, diarrhoea and complaints of abdominal pains. The evidence suggests that anxious children not only show larger physiological reactions to stress than other children, but also take longer to return to basal levels (Lader, 1980). Typically, research studies involving children make use of two or three measures of physiological activity, which are used to provide a basal level and an estimate of reactivity. The two systems which have been studied in most detail are electrodermal activity and cardiovascular functioning. Typical measures include skin conductance and rate of habituation to novel stimuli, heart rate, pulse rate and blood pressure. More complicated measures include muscle tremor, blood and urinary steroid levels and EEG activity (Venables, 1980).

Sociometry

While sociometry can properly be regarded as coming under the general heading of 'psychometric techniques', it is different from other approaches to the extent that the responses are gathered from the child's peer group and they do not include direct rating of the child's anxiety. There are several variations of technique in sociometric assessment (Williams & Gilmour, 1994; Hughes, 1988). The most popular method is peer nomination, which requires each child in a class or social group to choose several children (typically three) with respect to given criteria. Positive criteria are statements such as 'like the most' and 'would like to play with', and the negative criteria might be 'like the least' and 'would not like to play with'. Positive nomination scores from the group can be used to provide an estimate of popularity and peer acceptance, and negative nomination scores to reflect rejection. Creating structured scores allows recalculation of a social impact scale and more detailed classification systems – for example, 'neglected children' are those with relatively few positive and negative nominations, and 'controversial children' are those with a high social impact who are liked most by some children and liked least by others (Coie et al., 1982; Newcomb et al., 1993). The most common reason for social rejection appears to be aggressive behaviour, and there is evidence that aggressive, socially-rejected children are at risk for having later behavioural difficulties and conduct disorders. There is also a subgroup of rejected children who are socially withdrawn and do not show disruptive behaviour. Children in this latter category are at risk for bullying, and in some cases may develop later emotional disturbances, indicating the need for a more detailed assessment of their anxiety levels. Some socially-neglected children have low self-esteem and above-average anxiety levels, but current evidence suggests that this group is not more at risk than other children for later disturbances (Williams & Gilmour, 1994).

There are strong ethical reasons for insisting on the exercise of great care in the setting up of situations in which children are required to rate each other, whether for popularity or even for traits such as aggressiveness. Peer rating methods involving the use of Likert type scales are less obviously pejorative. The effect of the peer group on the individual is important, and for some children, their sociometric status changes when they move between groups.

Measurement of social attachment

Bowlby (1969) discussed attachment in terms of control systems theory. He drew attention to the evolutionary significance of attachment as a process designed to increase the chances of survival by ensuring proximity to the mother. From around the age of 8 months, babies seem to become aware of the strange and unfamiliar, and some react to separation by crying and other forms of distress.

Ainsworth devised the Strange Situation Test as a structured technique for measuring security of attachment in infants aged between 12 and 18 months. The procedure involves cumulative stress, with the infant experiencing two brief separations from the mother and interactions with a stranger in an unfamiliar room. Security of attachment is assessed from the infant's behaviour on the second reunion with the mother figure (Ainsworth et al., 1978). There have been numerous replications, and the procedure can be regarded as having achieved the status of a laboratory-based psychometric test.

Typically, around 65% of infants are classified as securely attached, showing some variation of greeting, approach behaviour or being comforted on the return of the mother, whether or not they were distressed during separation. Two categories of insecure attachment have been identified. Avoidant infants (around 20%) tend to ignore the mother rather than seek interaction on reunion, and resistant or anxious-ambivalent infants (around 10–15%) tend to mingle contact-seeking behaviour with angry and rejecting behaviour. The significance of these findings is that insecurely-attached infants appear to be more at risk for developing later emotional disturbance.

DSM-IV (American Psychiatric Association, 1994) identifies two anxiety conditions which, in different ways, reflect difficulties in social relationships and security of attachment. In 'reactive attachment of infancy or early childhood', there is a persistent failure to initiate or respond appropriately to social interaction. Some children show inhibited or ambivalent approach/avoidant behaviours, and others seem to make indiscriminate, shallow attachments to relative strangers. The category 'separation anxiety disorder' is characterised by excessive anxiety concerning separation from the home or those to whom the person is attached, the anxiety being beyond that which is expected for the child's developmental level. Such problems become especially troublesome when the child experiences difficulty in attending school. In assessing school refusal problems, it is important to identify the different influences of separation anxiety and fears associated with being in the school situation. Both conditions also need to be distinguished from truanting, a behaviour pattern where the child is not fearful of school but prefers to be elsewhere.

Klagsbrun and Bowlby (1976) devised a projective test to measure separation anxiety in children in the age range 4–7 years. The children are each shown a series of six photographs in which a child of the same gender is seen in a situation prior to experiencing possible separations. Three of the scenes are referred to as mild, for example parents going out for the evening, and three as more severe, for example the child's first day at school. The categorisation of responses identifies three areas of anxiety – generalised dread/anxiety ('something bad's going to happen'), fear (of ghosts, monsters, etc.) and somatic reaction ('he's getting a tummy ache'). The Seattle Version of the Separation Anxiety Test (Slough et al., 1988) provides an alternative set of test materials and a categorisation of responses which more closely reflects the Ainsworth classification of attachment. More recently, Wright et al. (1995) report on the use of a similar separation anxiety test with age-appropriate stimulus pictures for children of 8–12 years of age.

Concluding comments

Having taken account of the diversity of methods for assessing anxiety in children, we are reinforced in the view that care must be taken to avoid oversimplification of an exceedingly complex construct. Clinicians and researchers from widely different backgrounds acknowledge the importance of understanding anxiety as a key to understanding behaviour.

Before giving children tests, we need to ask questions about the purpose of the assessment. The choice of instruments is likely to be very different when the task is to compare groups of children, perhaps undergoing variations in treatment programmes, from that involving individual children being seen for a diagnostic assessment or being monitored during therapy. For comparing groups of children, administration of one or more of the self-report questionnaires is likely to provide a satisfactory estimate of trait-anxiety. The addition of a rating scale completed by parents or teachers should provide a degree of confirmation of the findings. In the detailed assessment of individual children, there may be an opportunity to include physiological measures, although the necessary equipment will not always be available in a clinic setting. An attempt should be made to obtain separate estimates of state-anxiety and trait-anxiety. Where there are concerns about a child's academic attainments, then a measure of test anxiety is called for.

The assessment of withdrawn and anxious children is always a challenge for the psychologist. In such cases, verbal responses cannot be relied on to reflect the child's cognitive abilities or feelings. Measurement of security of attachment, fear of separation, self-esteem and social integration all add to the overall picture. More so than in most assessment situations, the measurement of anxiety requires the use of several procedures. Ideally, an assessment should provide cross-validation between standardised psychometric tests and more informal estimates.

References

Achenbach, T.M. & Edelbrock, C.S. (1983) *Manual for Child Behavior Checklist and Revised Child Behavior Profile*, Burlington, VT: Department of Psychiatry, University of Vermont.

Ainsworth, M.D.S., Blehar, M., Waters, E. & Wal, S. (1978) *Strange Situation Behaviour of One Year Olds: Its Relation to Mother–Infant Interaction in the First Year and to Qualitative Differences in the Mother–Infant Attachment Relationships*, Hillsdale, NJ: Lawrence Erlbaum.

American Psychiatric Association (1994) *Diagnostic and Statistical Manual of Mental Disorders: Fourth Edition (DSM-IV)*, Washington, DC: American Psychiatric Association.

Asher, S.R., Hymel, S. & Renshaw, P.P. (1984) 'Loneliness in children', *Child Development*, 55, pp.1,456–64.

Battle, J. (1981) *Culture-Free SEI Self-Esteem Inventories for Children and Adults*, Austin, TX: Pro-ed.

Bellak, L. & Bellak, S. (1957) *The Thematic Apperception Test and the Children's Apperception Test in Clinical Use*, New York: Grune and Stratton.

Bowlby, J. (1969) *Attachment and Loss, Vol.1: Attachment*, New York: Basic Books.

Castaneda, A., McCandless, B. & Palermo, D. (1956) 'The children's form of the Manifest Anxiety Scale', *Child Development*, 27, pp.317–26.

Cattell, R.B. (1973) *Personality and Mood by Questionnaire*, San Francisco, CA: Jossey-Bass.

Cattell, R.B. & Scheier, I.H. (1961) *The Meaning and Measurement of Neuroticism and Anxiety,* Champaign, IL: Institute for Personality and Ability.

Coan, R.W. & Cattell, R.B. (1966) *Early School Personality Questionnaire,* Champaign, IL: Institute for Personality and Ability.

Coie, J.D., Dodge, K.A. & Coppotelli, H. (1982) 'Dimensions and types of social status: A cross-age perspective', *Developmental Psychology,* 18, pp.557–70.

Cummings, J.A. (1986) 'Projective drawings', in Knoff, H.M. (ed.) *The Assessment of Child and Adolescent Personality,* New York: Guilford Press.

Digman, J.M. (1990) 'Personality and structure: Emergence of the five factor model', *Annual Review of Psychology,* 41, pp.417–40.

Eysenck, H.J. (1970) *The Structure of Human Personality,* London: Methuen.

Eysenck, S.B.G. (1965) *Manual of the Junior Eysenck Personality Inventory,* London: University of London Press.

Eysenck, H.J. & Eysenck, S.B.G. (1975) *Manual of the Eysenck Personality Questionnaire,* London: Hodder and Stoughton.

Francis-Williams, J. (1968) *Rorschach with Children,* Oxford: Pergamon Press.

Gillis, J.S. (1980) *Child Anxiety Scale Manual,* Champaign, IL: Institute for Personality and Ability Testing.

Goldberg, L.R. (1993) 'The structure of phenotypic personality traits', *American Psychologist,* 48, pp.26–34.

Goyette, C.H., Conners, C.K. & Ulrich, R.F. (1978) 'Normative data on Revised Conners Parent and Teacher Rating Scales', *Journal of Abnormal Child Psychology,* 6, pp.221–36.

Greenspan, S. (1981) *The Clinical Interview of the Child,* New York: McGraw-Hill.

Hampson, S.E. (1995) 'The construction of personality', in Hampson, S.E. & Colman, A.M. (eds) *Individual Differences and Personality,* London: Longman, pp.20–39.

Hughes, J.N. (1988) *Cognitive Behaviour Therapy with Children in Schools,* New York: Pergamon Press.

Klagsbrun, M. & Bowlby, J. (1976) 'Responses to separation from parents: A clinical test for young children', *Projective Psychology,* 21(2), pp.7–26.

Koppitz, E.M. (1968) *Psychological Evaluation of Children's Human Figure Drawings,* New York: Grune and Stratton.

Lader, M.H. (1980) 'The psychophysiology of anxiety', in Van Praag, H.M., Lader, M.H., Rafaelsen, O.J. & Sacher, E.J. (eds) *Handbook of Biological Psychiatry Part II: Brain Mechanisms and Abnormal Behaviour – Psychophysiology,* New York: Guilford Press, pp.225–47.

McGuire, J. & Richman, N. (1988) *Preschool Behaviour Checklist,* Windsor: NFER-Nelson.

Newcomb, A.F., Bukowski, W.M. & Pattee, L. (1993) 'Children's peer relations: A meta-analytic of popular, rejected, neglected, controversial and average sociometric status', *Psychological Bulletin,* 113, pp.99–128.

Phillips, B.N. (1978) *School Stress and Anxiety: Theory Research and Intervention,* New York: Human Sciences Press.

Phillipson, H. (1973) *A Short Introduction to the Objects Relations Technique,* Windsor: NFER-Nelson.

Porter, R.B. & Cattell, R.B. (1963) *The Children's Personality Questionnaire,* Champaign, IL: Institute for Personality and Ability Testing.

Reynolds, C.R. & Paget, K.D. (1981) 'Factor analysis of the Revised Children's Manifest Anxiety Scale for blacks, whites, males and females with a national normative sample', *Journal of Consulting and Clinical Psychology*, 49(3), pp.352–9.

Reynolds, C.R. & Richmond, B.O. (1978) ' "What I think and feel": A revised measure of children's manifest anxiety', *Journal of Abnormal Child Psychology*, 6(2), pp.271–80.

Rutter, M., Tizard, J. & Whitmore, K. (1970) *Education, Health and Behaviour*, Harlow: Longman.

Sarason, I.G. (ed.) (1980) *Test Anxiety: Theory Research and Applications*, Hillsdale, NJ: Lawrence Erlbaum.

Sarason, S.B., Davidson, K.S., Lighthall, F.F., Waite, R.R. & Ruebush, B.K. (1960) *Anxiety in Elementary School Children: A Report of Research*, New York: John Wiley.

Slough, N.M., Goyette, M. & Greenberg, M.T. (1988) *Scoring Indices for the Seattle Version of the Separation Anxiety Test*, Seattle, WA: University of Washington.

Spielberger, C.D. (1966) 'Theory and research on anxiety', *Anxiety and Behaviour*, New York: Academic Press.

Spielberger, C.D., Gorsuch, R.L. & Lushene, R.E. (1970a) *Manual for the State-Trait Anxiety Inventory*, Palo Alto, CA: Consulting Psychologists Press.

Spielberger, C.D., Edwards, D.C., Montouri, J. & Lushene, R.E. (1970b) *The State-Trait Anxiety Inventory for Children*, Palo Alto, CA: Consulting Psychologists Press.

Stott, D.H. (1974) *Bristol Social Adjustment Guides Manual: The Social Adjustment of Children* (5th edn), London: Hodder and Stoughton.

Taylor, J.A. (1953) 'A personality scale of manifest anxiety', *Journal of Abnormal and Social Psychology*, 48, pp.285–90.

Venables, P.H. (1980) 'Automatic reactivity', in Rutter, M. (ed.) *Scientific Foundations of Developmental Psychiatry*, London: Heinemann Medical, pp.165–75.

Vizard, E. & Tranter, M. (1988) 'Helping young children to describe experiences of child abuse: General issues', in Bentovim, A., Elton, A., Hildebrand, J., Tranter, M. & Vizard, E. (eds) *Child Sexual Abuse Within the Family*, London: Wright.

Williams, T.R. & Gilmour, J.D. (1994) 'Annotation: Sociometry and peer relationships', *Journal of Child Psychiatry*, 35(6), pp.997–1,013.

Wright, J.C., Binney, V. & Smith, P. (1995) 'Security of attachment in 8–12 year olds: A revised version of the Separation Anxiety Test, its psychometric properties and clinical interpretation', *Journal of Child Psychiatry*, 36(5), pp.757–74.

6 Contribution of the psychodynamic approach

Susanna Isaacs Elmhirst

Those working in local authority child and adolescent mental health services have recently been issued with two official documents urging them to develop and maintain multidisciplinary services in this important field which is of great concern to everyone in this country, directly and indirectly: *Together We Stand* (NHS Health Advisory Service, 1995) and *The Health of the Nation* (Department of Health and Social Security, 1992). I welcome these publications because, although it is a number of years since I retired from the NHS, I have continued to work and teach in this field and have become very perturbed about the forces in our society working to undermine co-operation between colleagues, as well as about other aspects of decline in mental health provision which was our flourishing pride until only very recently.

In using this opportunity to describe a little of the growth of the formerly-named child guidance clinics (CGCs) and the importance of psycho-analysis in this growth, with examples which are mainly from one such mental health service for the young and their families, I run the risk of idealising the past and/or being accused of doing so, whereas my aim is to draw your attention to the fact that societies do not progress simply by jettisoning the past; rather, they move forward by learning from their successes and their failures. The study of history, including the personal histories of innumerable members of the species *Homo sapiens*, have taught us that certain fundamental aspects of our human nature change extremely slowly, if at all, so far as we yet know, and attention to a person's emotional and physical strengths and susceptibilities and their interrelationships at all ages and stages of life will not rapidly go out of date, if ever.

The child guidance movement and the extension of psycho-analytic techniques to children emerged simultaneously, and were vital partners in the development of what are now sometimes called the 'management' aspects of responses to the emotional problems of families, their individual members and the societies in which they live. In its usage, not only to delineate attention to the home and other facets of the young sufferers' immediate and extended environment but also as a controversial feature in current NHS affairs, the term 'management' is confusing and open to misunderstanding, even more now than when it was first used. So too was some of the language used from the start to describe the original aims of child guidance clinics.

Actually *guiding* children, with its implications of a leader and a led (or even the sighted leading the blind), was never the essential aim of interdisciplinary work in the clinics which grew to adolescence in the years after World War I and reached thriving maturity in response to the stimulus of the sufferings children endured during World War II. Both the teacher who wrote on yet another of a small girl's violent stories, 'Couldn't you sometimes write a nice story, Lucy?', and her mother, who rushed her up to a child psychiatric department for 'guidance', were of the hopeful opinion that children could be guided into developmental pathways which did not include fierce thoughts or deeds, however grossly inadequate, repressive or provocative their conditions of life and work turned out to be.

The particular plight of Lucy in this vignette about the solutions to her violent preoccupation, was, in part, very different, for a wider study of her situation revealed a homeless family with a father who, after a period of imprisonment for an offence to property, could only find low-paid warehouse work. His solution was to house his wife, Lucy and her siblings secretly in the attic of his employer's warehouse. The living conditions were materially sparse, warmth only achieved by huddling closely together at night, all the while under threat of discovery and punishment by eviction at best. These circumstances aroused great hatred and cruelty in Lucy, as well as fear and an urgent need for help, expressed by her stories.

Because the multidisciplinary CGC to which her mother turned, on the advice of a neighbour, was psychodynamically orientated, the family's beliefs, attempted solutions and failures were enquired into with sympathy and interest, but without being criticised or condoned. Understanding of Lucy's feelings was followed by a search for sources which might be altered in such a way as to lessen suffering and promote the natural healing which is so much a part of normal emotional health, especially in the young. Also borne in mind was the possibility of Lucy's emotional growth having been disturbed in such a way as potentially to interfere permanently and seriously with her satisfactions and maturation, an outcome which would have been thought to require individual psychotherapy for her. The assessment procedures in a genuinely multidisciplinary clinic have certain aspects in common with group or family approaches, while also bearing in mind the separate, differing, needs of each individual in a context where there is no essential discrepancy between the therapeutic rights of the individual and the group.

The particular multidisciplinary unit to which Lucy was taken developed directly out of studies begun during World War II. Many children were evacuated from the large cities under the threat of extensive bombing. Many of these children were much distressed and disturbed by this serious and complex attempt to protect their health and welfare. Many adults actively involved first reacted to the children's overt misery, to their antagonism to change, their bedwetting, delinquency and learning difficulties, and so on, with surprised disapproval and misunderstanding of their families of origin.

Later, many people became deeply interested in the children's difficulties, including D.W. Winnicott and his social work colleague, Clare, who later became his wife. In his post-World War II development, Winnicott in time founded and headed the first Department of Child Psychiatry in St Mary's Hospital, at No. 17 Paddington Green, which is where Lucy was brought in maternal agitation. Later in this chapter, I will take you back to 'Number Seventeen', which was one of the appreciative abbreviations it was known by. Meanwhile, we need to go further back still, to the part played by psychodynamically-achieved understanding in the conception and growth of the multidisciplinary child guidance movement.

Both the term 'psychodynamic' and embryonic activity in the field were imported from the USA – an encouraging example of international cross-fertilisation and co-operation. The concept found better conditions for growth in the UK than in the USA, partly due to the different impact of World War II in the UK, as I have indicated, and partly because child psycho-analysis at first developed predominantly in Europe, and was found to be a crucial ingredient of child guidance clinic development in the UK, in addition to other factors too complex to go into here.

Freud, having discovered the principles of free association and transference, which led him to increasing understanding of the child in all of us, took another fundamental step in the early 1900s. A woman who had herself benefited from psycho-analysis asked Freud's advice when her 5-year-old son developed a very limiting phobia of horses. Freud's response, which was revolutionary at that time, was to urge the father of 'little Hans' to encourage the child in talking freely about his feelings, and then to send a written account of these discussions to Freud, who gave further advice about how the problems raised should be discussed and responded to. Hans knew that Freud, called 'the Professor' in the family, was working to try to understand his fears. On one occasion, Hans and his father were discussing the boy's complex feelings towards his baby sister. He had feared that his mother would drop Hanna in the bath and kill her. But as they talked, Hans contributed that he himself had really wanted Hanna to die, 'because she screams so'. His father said: 'and then you'd be alone with Mummy. A good boy doesn't wish that sort of thing, though.'

Hans: (not yet 5) 'But he may THINK it.'
Father: 'But that isn't good.'
Hans: 'If he thinks it, it is good all the same, because you can write it to the Professor.' (Freud, 1955)

In Freud's words, 'the little patient summoned up courage to describe the details of his phobia . . . and take an active share in the analysis'. He went 'forging ahead', and 'the material brought up . . . far out-stripped our powers of understanding'.

Once, when asked why he laughed with relief at a factual answer to his question about where chickens come from, little Hans replied: 'because I like what you've told me'. Later, he responded in a similar way to the discovery of truths about himself.

The way in which Hans could accept awareness of unwelcome, unpleasant, even hostile, aspects of himself with immediate relief, and the fact that this knowledge also later led to the gradual disappearance of his severe symptom, increased Freud's interest in the opposition his adult parents could mount against understanding. At that time, Freud thought that no one but a father 'could possibly have prevailed on the child to make any such avowals'. However, he gradually changed that opinion, as his understanding of the interaction of unconscious responses to outer reality was steadily increased by his own work with adults and that of others with children, for he made no other forays himself into the psychoanalysis of children.

Psycho-analytic work with individual child patients was soon embarked on, more or less simultaneously, by Hugo Hellmuth, Anna Freud and Melanie Klein. In my view, Klein's expansion of the technique of free association was another stroke of genius, Freud's discovery of it having been the first.

Melanie Klein's training analysts were Ferenczi and Abraham. In the latter, she found a man whose interest in the role of the unconscious mind in mental life had led him to the analysis of adults suffering from manic-depressive illnesses, and thus to the importance of oral fantasies and delusions, findings also relevant to less disordered but none the less suffering patients. Klein (1932) was freed in her analysis to draw on her personal and professional knowledge of the fact that in small children, 'action, which is more primitive than thought or words, forms the chief part of its behaviour'.

She formed the original theory that the relative lack of verbal free association in children need not be a barrier to psycho-analysing them, because in an analytic setting, a child's use of toys in undirected play, considered in conjunction with their spontaneous speech, song, sounds and movements, can be taken as exactly equivalent to the free association of adults. She therefore began to give her child patients small, simple toys to use in their sessions with her. She made no restrictions on what the child should do with these materials, other than that they should not be used with physical destructiveness against the patients themselves, the analyst or the room and its contents. She also, of course, allowed children the same privileges as adult patients, who were, and are, encouraged to *say* whatever thoughts or feelings occurred to them, secure in the knowledge that confidentiality was guaranteed and punishment, moral and physical, eschewed. To this verbal *carte blanche* and open-minded scrutiny of the details of the child's use of the toys was added detailed attention to their non-verbal sounds, songs and movements.

Using this technique, Klein found that children reveal great anxieties, and that, to some degree, these can be relieved by interpretation, just as they can with adults. The child patients with whom Klein started her psycho-analytic career were very young and very disturbed, children whom she found to be paralysed in their emotional growth by fears of all manner of attacks. Verbalising their fears to the children – which were, in the analysis, at first revealed as fear of attack by the analyst – gave them relief, which led to feelings of gratitude and an appetite for more (Klein, 1932). In other words, interpretation of the negative transference led to the development of a positive transference.

Klein first started seeing children psychodynamically in their own homes. She soon found that their anxieties about revealing conscious and unconscious 'forbidden' fears and furies in such intimate proximity to their parents and other caretakers, towards whom and by whom such feelings had originally been evoked, were so powerful an inhibitory force as to halt or limit progress. Seen elsewhere, in a relatively anonymous room equipped for children to move and play in, their more rapid and sustained progress confirmed her theory and increased her knowledge (see also Isaacs Elmhirst, 1988). From these discoveries came the development of an effective therapeutic method of approach to childhood emotional disorders – the psycho-analysis of children, which in turn was an essential ancestor of all psychodynamic child 'play' therapies and an important informant of dynamic family and group therapies. So too was the improved technique for the pyscho-analysis of adults which, in Klein's hands, led to the burgeoning of a group of psycho-analysts as remarkable and influential as Freud's original brood.

From Klein's adaptation of Freud's technique to children also came a greater understanding of the great differences there can at times be between the outward reality of the people mainly involved in a child's care and education and the representations of them in the child's conscious and unconscious mind. As the interest in these findings spread psycho-analytically and to other areas of work with children and adults, Freud's perception that the first ego is a body ego was increasingly substantiated. Furthermore, it became clearer that in adults with thought disorders, persistence or recrudescence of concrete thinking is a problem only partially resolved in development from infancy, where such experiences of 'feelings as things' was found to be a normal precursor to, and accompaniment of, the development of a capacity for abstract mental representation, which is the basis for verbal communication, with its subtleties and sophistications.

To return to Winnicott, who was a paediatrician to whom many babies and young children were brought as patients, his studies furthered our awareness of the normal psychosomatic responsiveness of all infants, as well as of the pathological variations found, some of which can actually prove fatal. They also opened up areas of interrelatedness from earliest infancy onwards, in particular the dependency of babies on their mothers, and the complexities of mother–infant interaction. So deep was Winnicott's interest that it was an important source of his decision to change specialities and, in time, to become a psycho-analyst of adults and children.

He studied in particular the way in which many babies became intensely attached to some part of their inanimate world, such as a rug or soft toy, and invest them with important powers. He called these infantile creations 'transitional objects' (Winnicott, 1951). His perception of their emotional importance was a stroke of genius. Among other results from the work this stimulated has been greater understanding of the developmental importance of relationships between an infant's perceptions of internal and external happenings, sometimes summarised as the infant's perceptions of, and need to differentiate between, 'fantasy and reality' or even 'fact and fantasy'.

Winnicott's oft-repeated phrase, 'there is no such thing as a baby', means, by implication, that there is no such thing as a baby without a mother (or mother-substitute), but also that there is no such thing as a mother (or surrogate) without a baby. He was specifically speaking of emotional dependency, while his meaning was also consciously and deliberately rooted in awareness of biological reality. No human offspring can survive without appropriate nourishment from outside; nor can anyone be conceived except by the union of male and female gametes.

We need now to consider another psycho-analyst central to our understanding of the human mind, of its development, and thus of how to further or hinder its maturation and creativity. I refer to W.R. Bion, arguably the greatest of all those psycho-analysed by Melanie Klein. He did not work directly with children, but in the course of his psychoanalytic study of adults, in groups and individuals with psychotic disorders of thought, he perceived and formulated what he summarised as 'the threeness' of the human mind (Bion, 1961, 1962).

His theory was that the human is born with many 'pre-conceptions'. When any of these pre-conceptions meets ('mates' with) a 'realisation', the outcome is a mental 'concept'. These concepts are essential elements of thought, a capacity for which is a basic source of the strength and flexibility of the human mind. It was that aspect of the mind to which little Hans was referring in his own way when he said: 'But it is good, because then you can write it to the Professor', with the implication that Freud could and would think about Hans's thoughts, including his destructive thoughts. He quickly learnt that Freud would not be too fearful to read them, see them, and also be able to return thinkable thoughts to Hans's father, and thence to the little boy himself.

Such interactions are, in Bion's view, essential in the human's development away from concrete and magical beliefs in their own mental powers, or those of others, toward an awareness of the capacity of the more mature mind to abstract meaning in a way which offers freedom for individuality and escape from the tyrannical rule of the 'omnipotence of thoughts' which is inevitable, and indeed, at times, of much value in infancy.

One important aspect of the interaction between a person and their environment, from earliest infancy onwards, is the use of projection as a method of ridding the mind of painful experiences. One root of such a mechanism is the belief that experiences are concrete, to be got rid of and/or taken in as desired. The predominance of that belief in infants leads, under normal circumstances, to the development of a capacity to differentiate good from bad and safe from dangerous experiences. Such differentiation is a step forward from the undifferentiated, omnipotent confusion of self and object. Winnicott called transitional objects the 'first-not-me' objects, which are also not mother and, in my opinion, contain elements of what in later development would be recognised as delusional distortions (Isaacs Elmhirst, 1980).

The fact that such beliefs can predominate in psychotic states in later childhood and adult life is illustrated by a 10-year-old boy who was observed in hospital to be banging one side of his head vigorously with his hand. When asked if he could say why he was doing this, he promptly explained that he had some nasty thoughts in his head which he wanted to get out of it. However, the comment of a young girl whose father would not permit any toys or 'nonsense play' in the cot, 'my Daddy didn't seem to want me ever to have been a baby', is a revealing parallel to the small boy who assured me that he, personally, had never been a baby, he'd never been younger than 4 – and that was evidently almost unbelievably frighteningly near the horrors of infancy as *he* had experienced them (Isaacs Elmhirst, 1981).

All three of these vignettes are from work with children who could speak and understand spoken speech. Thus they illustrate how complex and sophisticated their mental growth already was, as well as showing that they experienced thoughts in two different ways and were able to communicate them simultaneously in two very different ways. Thinking is dependent on the creation and use of concepts, mentioned earlier as being abstracted from the union of a pre-conception and a realisation.

Among the great opportunities opened up by the achievement of abstract conceptualisation are the differentiation of physical from emotional reality, of the imagination from delusional and hallucinatory misperceptions. Thus do humans become able, even as young babies, to accept that they can feel very hostile to those they most love and are grateful to. Acquisition of such awareness is painful, the pain of regret and sadness about the fate of loved ones in the imagination. From such regret and sadness springs the urge to repair the sources of life itself, to free loved ones to live their own lives in imagination, and to some extent in the world beyond the control of the imagination. The actual fulfilment in real-life achievement of loving, reparative, creative and respectful relationships and activities is both difficult and satisfying. The first steps of infantile learning about the real possibilities which lie in human interrelationships are taken within the family. Practical love, concerned protection and the encouragement of appropriate moves to independence all require continuity of physical care and emotional climate.

To a greater or lesser extent, the growth of any infant is impaired by many interruptions of emotional or physical sustenance, with physically-expressed hate in the form of physical or sexual abuse being especially damaging. In the usual 'good-enough' family, infants are allowed the time and the circumstances in which they can achieve a stable enough, benign enough inner world of memory and imagination to be able to carry it with them on to substitute care, which, if it is also at least adequate, will increase their knowledge of the variability of trustworthy adults. Thus transition from infant daycare to nursery education, and so on, can be achieved satisfyingly, though not without the effort of overcoming anxieties and inner opposition. That there may be overt or more subtle opposition in the adults involved is a pivotal area of study in inter-disciplinary work with families.

Parents, or teachers, who unconsciously view children as more or less intractably mindless (be they white, black, male or female) *are* depriving the children, although they would find it extremely hard to let themselves become aware of such an unwelcome, and unwelcoming, even abusive, attitude. Yet change and adaptation are human capacities, and those involved in a multidisciplinary approach to children and families, within clinics and within wider society, have to be constantly on the alert for any evidence of prejudicial attitudes within themselves. Often, this is easier in a clinic, where even the most difficult parents, the most resistant to change, bring their children, and thus themselves, spontaneously in search of help in a setting where colleagues operate to help each person concerned, including each other. Therapeutic work with a single mother whose son correctly observed 'she doesn't bear me no mind' presented no easy task. But it would have been impossible if she had been approached as 'the cause' of the child's fear of developing and revealing a mind of his own.

Fortunately, many who have been subject to overt or more subtle forms of prejudicial implications of blame are very sensitive to the opposite attitude of open-minded enquiry which characterises the psychodynamic approach. The concentration and cultivation of such an attitude, especially in multidisciplinary child guidance clinics, can lead to a working relationship between the staff and the families with whom they are concerned. This is illustrated by the response of a small girl to a new social worker on a home visit to try and help her anxious and ashamed parents visit the clinic, which the child and her grandmother had braved and found more than safe, found it to be a positively helpful working unit. The child patient knew the clinic as a source of sympathetic and reassuring enquiry. In her mind, she extended this quality to all at the clinic, known or unknown. Thus the visiting worker seemed naturally trustworthy to her, so that her frightened parents were much encouraged by their child's request of the visitor, 'May I sit on your lap, Paddington Green?', and by the social worker's encouraging but not provocatively effusive agreement to such a request.

It is often wrongly supposed that the psychodynamic approach necessarily involves acquiescence in, tolerance of, even encouragement of, freedom to enact whatever wishes may arise, be they greedy, intrusive or more obviously aggressive. The roots of such misconceptions lie in the incomplete differentiation in many adults between feeling and doing, between verbal expression and the power to override the limits of reality. Of course, it is not true that 'words can never hurt', for words can indeed cause pain, as can unspoken attitudes. But words and fantasies expressed symbolically in other ways cannot kill, maim, break and enter in physical reality. That fact is easy enough to put firmly down on paper, yet once established, it is still no easy task to reinstate it as the predominant view of the human mind when personally affronted or confronted by adults who have physically and/or sexually abused the children in their care.

The emotional stresses and strains of work with troubled children and their families are very great, and make the work of interdisciplinary co-operation within a clinic very hard but very rewarding. One of the rewards for such clinics or departments is the capacity to influence the whole area in which they are centred. But change takes time, and learning takes time, including the processes of not being able to learn, or of un-learning, which are the cause of so much suffering, perhaps especially obviously in school-age children. In the modern world, it is hard to counter the widespread belief that speed and numerically quantifiable results are signs of progress. Such a task is made harder when confused by misunderstanding of the vital interactions of learning, and con-structive use of such acquired treasure and thus the acquisition of further knowledge and the skills to use and increase it.

In early life, play is the child's equivalent of work; not only can it be pleasurable and satisfying, but it is *needed*, as is work of some kind, for all adults. The word 'depression' crept into daily English usage in the 1930s, recognised as a consequence of unemployment for a whole society and its individual members. If it is indeed true that the level of violence is increasing now in our society, as well as its recognition, then we are in a worrying vicious circle, for the violent need restraint, understanding and appropriate occupation, with opportunities for creative not destructive expression.

It can be very discouraging for the staff of multidisciplinary units if they set themselves, or are set, unattainably high standards, which mean they are not given official appreciation of both the immediate and long-term importance of combining the relief of present suffering with the formulation and implementation of a long-term, open-ended plan for the family as a whole. Such realistic plans need to be rooted in assessment of the needs, capabilities and unknowns inherent in even the smallest family group.

One source of the irreplaceable role of psychiatrists in such assessments and 'management' plans is their relative inability to lose sight of certain fundamental facts. I refer to the fact that the practice of medicine, and training for it, repeatedly confronts its members with the real destructibil-ity of human life, by death or irreparable physical damage. I refer also to the painfully-acquired knowledge that treatment can cause harm despite conscious intentions that it will do the opposite, as well as to the axiom that treatment should be instituted *after* diagnosis (i.e. assessment) and with as clear a picture as possible of the prognosis, the prospects, for each patient or group of patients (i.e. sufferers).

The importance of communication in the service of the search for understanding cannot be overestimated, and has been vividly illustrated for me by what may seem to some people to be a paradox, which is that a well-running NHS and/or local authority multidisciplinary assessment centre for patients can provide an incomparably better service for young people and their families than can the most experienced and expert clinician conducting private consultations. In the case of psychosomatic disorders, close co-operation between such a centre and the paediatric and GP services is even more necessary. Of course, communication can, and often must, be achieved and maintained by individuals, but there is the added reassurance of geographical propinquity, which is so beneficial and worth striving for in work with families in trouble.

The particular technical difficulties of psycho-analysis and psycho-therapy often mean that such forms of treatment cannot be offered in a clinic, any more than can specialised medical or surgical care, limited task-orientated teaching, and so on. Also, there will always be a need for some residential assessment and treatment centres of various types, whatever the prevailing winds of fashion may dictate.

The wider educational influence of interdepartmental co-operation is illustrated by the situation of another very young child, receiving once-weekly psychotherapy for faecal retention and overflow while her single mother met with a social worker in the hope of relief from at least her more delusional fears about the dangers of not having a daily bowel movement. The child, Nancy, made good progress until she only soiled when there was an interruption in the regular pattern of weekly sessions. Such interruptions were mainly predictable: even a female medical psycho-analyst must take a holiday sometimes or sometimes gets the 'flu.

During the course of therapy, the little girl came to feel and express anger, despite her belief that in doing so she would cause disaster and be disastrously punished. She once seriously believed that she had caused a thunderstorm which erupted just as a session ended. It was a session in which she had played with soap and water, which she daringly confided were really 'wee-wee and pooh'. My survival and non-punitive efforts to understand her fears and feelings and verbalise them for her were deeply relieving and encouraging.

Pondering this led me to the decision that when there was the next holiday interruption, I would write a careful message in the notes to whichever doctor was on call, to be read in the event that the agitated mother brought up her daughter in search of an enema to wash out her bad, dangerous, retained faeces. My written suggestion was that the doctor on call reassure the mother and ask her to return with Nancy after 24 hours if the retention persisted. I knew that *en route* to the hospital outpatient department, mother and child had to pass the house in which I worked when not away. I surmised that the sight of the intact house and the fact of a colleague reading what I had written would, in and of themselves, be sufficiently reassuring to Nancy unconsciously to release her to have a normal, spontaneous bowel movement, for she was clearly not consciously or deliberately withholding her faeces in order to worry her mother, nor to provoke the dreaded intrusion of an enema.

In other sessions, she had revealed similar fantasies of having explosively extruded her father, full of wee-wee and pooh, from the family, her and mother as pure as soap and water but at risk of violent retribution and robbery. Sometimes, even an enema could be reassuring, in that she had so far survived each one. But she suffered awful fears before and during their administration, losing all good memories as she lost control. In part, her fears were of being robbed of all her good feelings, and then violently, explosively, left as full of badness.

As regards the next holiday break in therapy, all went as predicted, in that the small patient's faecal retention *did* recur in my absence, and her mother *did* take her up to the hospital, walking past the Department of Child Psychiatry in the process. In the outpatient department, the doctor in charge *did* read my note, and the little girl *did*, later that day, spontaneously defecate.

Mother was delighted, immediately reporting it to her social worker when treatment resumed after the holiday. But my small patient said nothing to me spontaneously. However, I had cause to comment on the holiday happenings, of which she first claimed she had no memory, and then said: 'Oh yes, I saw a doctor who could read.'

I hope some of the wider implications of this vignette are evident. It may seem exaggerated to claim that child and adolescent mental health services are of importance in the growth and maintenance of a civilised society; none the less, it is my considered opinion. For such services not only have to have active staff co-operation within the clinic, but to widen it to schools, social services, police and other community-based activities, which are all of significance to families. To support this contention, which I think is supported by the two publications mentioned at the start of this chapter, I will end with an extract from a book about the collapse of standards in a country which has acquired and maintained civilised standards in many areas. American psycho-analyst Leo Rangell wrote, in *The Mind of Watergate*:

I have not presumed to answer the question of 'how' to make man change in the right direction. It is enough that I describe as much as I can of the 'what' and gingerly try to approach the 'whys'. If the question of 'how' then becomes uppermost to others I hope they will take it from there. The psycho-analyst can contribute (knowledge of) the forces which operate in the unconscious, but for an approach to solutions, a team effort is necessary – with humanists and social scientists, psychiatrists and theologians and even the physical and biological scientists joining toward a common goal. (Rangell, 1980, p.304)

References

Bion, W.R. (1961) *Experiences in Groups*, London: Tavistock Publications.

Bion, W.R. (1962) *The Elements of Psycho-Analysis*, London: Heinemann.

Department of Health and Social Security (1992) *The Health of the Nation: Strategy for Health in England*, London: HMSO.

Freud, S. (1955) 'Analysis of a phobia in a 5 year old boy "Little Hans" ', in Strachey, J. (ed.) *The Standard Edition of the Complete Psychological Works of Sigmund Freud*, Vol.X: 1909, London: Hogarth Press, pp.5–21.

Isaacs Elmhirst, S. (1980) 'Transitional objects in transition', *International Journal of Psycho-Analysis*, 61, p.367.

Isaacs Elmhirst, S. (1981) 'Bion and babies', in *Do I Dare Disturb the Universe?*, Caesura Press, p.83.

Isaacs Elmhirst, S. (1988) 'The Kleinian setting for child analysis', *International Review of Psycho-Analysis*, 15.

Klein, M. (1932) 'The psycho-analysis of children', in Thorner, H.A. (1975) *The Writings of Melanie Klein* (Vol.II), London: Hogarth Press and International Psycho-Analytical Library, pp.3–293.

NHS Health Advisory Service (1995) *Together We Stand: Child and Adolescent Mental Health*, London: HMSO, Department of Health, Science and Education.

Rangell, L. (1980) *The Mind of Watergate: An Exploration of the Compromise of Integrity*, New York and London: W.W. Norton.

Winnicott, D.W. (1951) 'Transitional objects and transitional phenomena', *International Journal of Psycho-Analysis*, 36.

7 Cognitive behavioural therapy

Mary Ellis

Although all the necessary research work to classify anxiety disorders in children is not yet complete (compare World Health Organisation, 1992, and American Psychiatric Association, 1994) and there have been insufficient controlled studies of psychotherapeutic or pharmacological treatment, it is essential to offer treatment to children whose fears and anxieties are persistent and disabling. Fears and anxiety are normal and necessary from an evolutionary point of view. Separation anxiety has been observed in many species, as well as in humans, and serves the purpose of maintaining the contact between mother and offspring when dangers are unpredictable and the possibility of getting lost great.

The evolution of fears in humans from infancy to adulthood follows a developmental path which would certainly increase the likelihood of survival in a primitive environment. Earliest fears are of sudden loss of physical contact (being dropped) and of loud noises, followed by distress at separation from caregivers and fear of strangers, later fear of falling, fear of animals and of the dark. These are followed in middle childhood, as the child's experiences and cognitive abilities develop, by performance anxieties and interpersonal anxieties.

The factor structure of the Fear Survey Schedule for Children (Ollendick et al., 1989) reflects these fears, even though the order does not follow them:

- Factor 1 – failure and criticism.
- Factor 2 – the unknown.
- Factor 3 – minor injury and small animals.
- Factor 4 – danger and death.
- Factor 5 – medical fears.

This schedule has now been used in various countries and continents, and children's fears have been found to be remarkably similar, with variations

113

more likely at older ages – 11 years and older – and thought to be culturally determined (Dong et al., 1994).

Consistency of fears over time was found to be greatest at the extreme levels. Children who reported the highest fear levels at younger ages were more likely to have high fear scores two years later (Spence & McCathie, 1993).

Research shows that temperament contributes to reactions to feared situations. There are individual differences in fearful responses and behavioural inhibition which are characteristic and are consistent from infancy to childhood (Kagan et al., 1988). Correlations between children's fear scores on the Fear Survey Schedule for Children-Revised (FSSC-R – Ollendick, 1983) and scores of anxiety measured by the Revised Children's Manifest Anxiety Scale (RCMAS) are highly significant (Ollendick et al., 1991).

The contribution of genetics is not yet fully understood (Stevenson et al., 1992; Thapar & McGuffin, 1995). However, in clinical practice, fearful parents are certainly overrepresented in families of children referred with anxiety disorders. Indeed, DSM-III-R (American Psychiatric Association, 1987) stated that neglected children are underrepresented among those with separation anxiety. The families of children with overanxious disorder tend to be small, in the upper socio-economic groups, and they tend to exhibit concern about achievement even when the child functions at an adequate or superior level. Anxiety disorders are also said to be more common in mothers of these children.

A cognitive behavioural approach is based on the idea that, in the modern world, it is not always the event which gives rise to our emotional responses, but our appraisal of the event, and that over time, we build up schemata of the world into which events fit and which affect our reactions to events. These schemata may be adaptive, in which case they will be flexible, or maladaptive, in which case they are likely to be rigid. They also become unconscious, rather as we are eventually no longer aware of every movement involved in walking or driving a car. If schemata are maladaptive, then the behaviours which follow the activation of the schemata are likely to be maladaptive.

Cognitive behavioural therapy (CBT) addresses the automatic thoughts and images, which may activate the schemata, by modifying them, and so the therapy helps to modify behavioural consequences. These are also addressed more directly by behavioural experiments which are part of the therapy, and these in turn lead to modification of automatic thoughts, images and schemata. The great advantage of using this approach with children is that they are still in the process of developing schemata, which are often much less rigid than those of adults with anxiety disorders.

Beck (1976) suggests that anxious people systematically overestimate the danger in situations. Children, of course, do not know how to assess the dangerousness of situations or the relevance of the feelings they experience, for example feeling as though they cannot breathe, or having a tummy ache. They gradually build up a picture of the world by presenting adults with emotions and feelings and experience for feedback. If parents or carers respond with anxious concern to all their approaches, their own anxiety and arousal is maintained.

Arousal and anxiety in the face of danger is, of course, normal. We have inherited an anxiety programme from our evolutionary past designed to protect us from danger. This includes the following:

- changes in autonomic arousal to prepare for fight, flight or fainting;
- inhibition of ongoing behaviour (compare increased rates of anxiety disorder in inhibited children and relatives with uninhibited groups);
- scanning the environment for danger. (adapted from Hawthorn et al., 1993, p.54)

The overactivation of this anxiety programme can lead to long periods away from school or long admissions to hospital, and many investigations, medications and, at worst, operations.

For the reasons above, and for the pragmatic reason that it is often effective and speedy, cognitive behavioural therapy should be considered as the first-line approach to anxiety disorders in children.

Cognitive behavioural therapy for children with anxiety disorders

In order to engage the child and family in therapy, the central tenets of CBT need to be conveyed: *it is our interpretation of events, rather than the events themselves, which give rise to distressing feelings and maladaptive behaviours.* This sequence can be altered by child, family and therapist co-operating together in the use of certain cognitive and behavioural techniques. Progress is continually assessed by all the participants.

Engaging the child involves explaining and demonstrating how they will learn to have control over the unpleasant feelings, while being able to engage in all age-appropriate activities, behaviours, school, sport and social activities. For instance, *anxiety* and *excitement* are very similar in terms of physiological reactions – for example, increased heart rate, flushing, 'gut reactions', sweaty palms, and so on – but are very different in how we are thinking about or picturing the future event. This can be demonstrated in the clinic, and may constitute the first behavioural experiment in which the child is engaged.

Assessment

This is of great importance, lasts from the first meeting until the end of therapy, and is integral to it. A full psychiatric history is an excellent starting point. Parents and children often volunteer information which can be used for more data-led assessment, for example: 'it always seems to happen first thing in the morning before school', or 'before a particular lesson' or 'at bedtime'. It is then easy to focus on one such event and elicit a detailed description of a recent occurrence:

- Where did it happen, and when?
- What physical symptoms were experienced?
- What thoughts/pictures did the child (and the parents) have?
- What did the child do (i.e. behaviours)?
- What did the parents do (i.e. behaviours)?
- Are there other triggers, other situations where the symptoms are likely to occur?
- What do the symptoms prevent the child from doing?
- What does the child or family do to avoid these unpleasant feelings, etc., happening?
- What things make the symptoms worse, or better?
- What makes it easier or more difficult for the family or the teacher to cope?
- What possible explanations for the symptoms does the family have?
- How did it all start? How has it progressed?
- What have they done to change things?

Sharing the rationale for CBT and assessment go hand in hand, and include assessment of suitability for this treatment approach. Parents who remain convinced, for whatever reason, of a different explanation, or who feel blamed, or who find it hard to join in a co-operative venture with the therapist and child, will not be able to support this form of treatment. They may have had medication themselves and prefer that approach, or been unable to engage in CBT for their own anxiety problems (for instance, one father wanted his daughter helped, but was convinced and kept reiterating that 'There is no cure for generalised anxiety.'). It may still be possible to help the child using some of the elements of CBT in conjunction with other treatments, but the parents' views should be respected.

Assessing the child

There has now been research in several countries into the fears and worries of children between the ages of $4\frac{1}{2}$ and adolescence (Stevenson-Hinde & Shouldice, 1995). The research shows that:

- At the extreme, the fears are likely to be most persistent.
- While the content of the fears changes over time, they are present at all ages.
- Maternal rating of children's levels of fear are not always consistent with those of the children themselves, particularly boys.
- There is significant correlation between fears and anxiety.

It is therefore important to spend time alone with the child, or if they are too young or too fearful, at least to elicit their fears, their physical symptoms and their view of the behaviour the two produce, as well as eliciting this from the parents. When encouraged to share their fears and helped with the use of age-appropriate toys, forms, drawings and so on, children are as informative as adults. With the youngest children, it is helpful to have the parents present, as they will become co-therapists. With slightly older children who are already attending school, and so have to be able to function away from parents, some time alone is helpful. It prepares them to become competent to handle their own worries as therapy progresses. The ability to feel in some control helps to develop their self-confidence. From the age of 10, children enjoy being treated as an important partner in the assessment and planning of therapy. If forms are tailored to their capabilities, they seem to overcome fears of the therapy quickly. From the age of 14, it is possible to use adult methods of record-keeping, such as panic diaries or forms for recording thoughts, etc. During the assessment, they are introduced to these, and their reactions used as part of the assessment.

For each child it is necessary to elicit:

- physical symptoms most often experienced (with the child's particular words for these symptoms), for example palpitations, difficulty breathing, abdominal pains, difficulty thinking;
- images/thoughts that go with these symptoms/feelings;
- frightening images/thoughts that the child has;
- anything that the child does to stop the unpleasant symptoms/ feelings or images/thoughts.

Record-keeping

This is an important element of the CBT approach. It helps everyone – therapist, parents and child – to assess progress. It also means that discussions take place around thoughts and feelings transposed from 'inside', where they are hard to understand and therefore 'powerful', to pieces of paper which can be shared and changed together. For children, the scales have to be adapted to be age-appropriate. Visual analogue scales are the easiest to understand. Understandable names need to be found for body sensations and added to any scales already in use. Pictures are best used for feelings in younger children. For instance, one can use sticky labels and the names and characters of the Mr Men and Little Miss series, for example Miss Happy, Mr Messy, Mr Mean, Mr Fussy, Mr Muddle, Mr Grumpy, Mr Quiet, Mr Worry (Hargreaves, 1990). Children sometimes find it easier to describe or draw the *picture* they see in their own minds when they are anxious, rather than *thoughts* (so do some adults).

Treatment plans and aims

The general aims of CBT are to reduce fears and anxiety to comfortable proportions under the control of the child, to reduce maladaptive behaviours, especially avoidance, and enhance the range of adaptive behaviours available to the child. The specific aims may be, for example, to bring panic attacks under control, to sleep in their own bed, to bring tummy aches before school under control, and so on. They must be important to the child and to the parents. Once one aim has been achieved, one progresses to the next, until the child and family are satisfied. Deciding together is part of the CBT approach and keeps it co-operative, what Beck et al. (1979) described as 'collaborative empiricism', which, of course, also keeps the family engaged.

Individual sessions, which may take place weekly or fortnightly, have a relatively set pattern:

1 discuss the previous week;
2 discuss homework, once CBT is under way;
3 the family decide on the aims for the present session;
4 teach any skills which may be needed – for example, relaxation, visualisation;
5 decide on record-keeping;
6 include the parents in helping with record-keeping and homework;
7 ask the child (and parents, if appropriate) to rate the session on a visual analogue scale.

Let us look in detail at the elements of an individual session.

Discussion about the previous week

Anything that may have occurred during the previous week which the child or family consider to be important and wish to share is elicited. Obviously, one wants to hear about any events which gave rise to considerable anxiety or any time the child was unable to do something because of their fears and anxieties. It is important to accept in a neutral way anything which the child or the parents share. The therapist must accept any explanations of what happened as a hypothesis, because the rest of the therapy will depend upon this.

Discussion of homework, once CBT is under way

This is obviously an important element of any session. It is equally important to know what was successful and what was unsuccessful, and to try to understand with the child, and if appropriate with the family, the reasons for either.

Deciding on the aims for the present session

If possible, these should arise from either of the first two steps, but of course, if there is some other matter which is very much in the forefront of the mind of the child or the parents, then that should be accepted. It is important at this point to elicit all the elements of this particular aim. For instance, if it is that the child should sleep in their own bed, it is important to elicit any fears or anxieties which are allied to this, such as fear of the dark, ghosts, and so on. It would also be important to elicit the physical symptoms which result from the child thinking or imagining what might happen in the dark, and also what behaviours they now resort to in order to avoid the discomfort. It would almost certainly be important to break down this aim into several smaller steps, starting with control over the frightening thoughts and images and the uncomfortable feelings that they lead to.

Teaching any skills which may be needed

The first stage in teaching any skills which might be needed to help the child to bring their thoughts/images and reactions under control might be to encourage the child to share their thoughts or images, either verbally or by drawing them. This could lead to discussion of what would help make them less frightened of ghosts, for instance imagining that they had secret strengths such as Batman might have. Since the discussion in the session is likely to produce symptoms of anxiety and uncomfortable feelings, the therapist can go on to using relaxation or visualisation techniques in the session to help the child deal with the symptoms. Homework would then be to continue to use the techniques at home as well as within the session, to the point where the child can think of being in the dark alone without discomfort.

Deciding on record-keeping

The therapist and child and family can decide between them how to keep a record, both of any practice the child does and the effect it has on minimising symptoms. The method of keeping records should be as simple as possible, and as pleasurable as possible for the child. It will then contribute to the child's feeling of competence.

Including parents in helping with record-keeping and homework

Including the parents will, of course, act as reinforcement, but they must be helped to be supportive and not add a further anxiety to the child's current anxieties, for example that it has not 'performed well enough' for the therapist.

Asking the child (and parents, if appropriate) to rate the session on a visual analogue scale

The last part of the session is to rate the session itself, which is most easily done on the visual analogue scale. This provides feedback for the therapist, which is of great importance and also helps to keep the therapist, the child and the parents as equal partners in this enterprise. Great care must be given to the choice of homework, which must be within the child's ability, be explained clearly and have the parents' agreement and support. Child and parents are asked to feed back to the therapist what it is they have understood that they will be doing as homework. This helps the therapist to be sure that if the homework is not done, it will not be because the task has not been understood. Parents and, where appropriate, the child should be part of assessing the homework and the progress.

Therapist

It is most important that the therapist maintains a neutral stance towards any information the child and family provide, and to the answers to any questions that the therapist poses. This can be done easily if the therapist remembers that everything can be thought of as a hypothesis. Each hypothesis can then be tested by asking questions, such as:

- 'Do you think that is the only way to explain what happened?'
- 'Do you think that your friend/brother/sister (etc.) would explain it in the same way?'
- 'Do you think that anyone could do as well in the test as you would like?'
- 'Do you think that everyone will always like you, agree with you (etc.)?'
- 'Do you think that you are thinking of all the things that you could do in the situation?'

Difficulty breathing, the second most common fear on the FSSC-R (Ollendick et al., 1991), or feeling faint with pins and needles, are good examples to take. If the child or family find it difficult to think of other explanations except catastrophic medical ones for this experience, it is possible to demonstrate by asking the child to hyperventilate in the session, in order that this hyperventilation can explain the symptoms and also, of course, how to deal with them very simply. The parents, too, can have this demonstrated to them, which will increase their confidence.

Avoidance

This maladaptive behaviour is the most difficult for parents and child to change. It is an inevitable human reaction, and is appropriate in some situations. However, an overanxious child will be using it in preference to other strategies, and almost certainly by the time child and family are referred to psychiatric services, the parents will be colluding. They are, of course, doing this out of love for their child, and need to be helped to accept that short-term distress leads to long-term resolution and progress. This is often best done by eliciting all the positive coping skills that the child already has. If one then devises exercises in which parents and child separately predict what will happen and how great the discomfort for the child will be when they carry such an exercise out, at least two things follow. One is that child and parents both find that they overestimate the amount of distress and difficulty that the child will experience, and secondly, they underestimate the capabilities of the child when a different strategy has been suggested and possibly rehearsed.

Many of the strategies which are used to help the family overcome the avoidance are behavioural and well known. However, introducing the element of prediction produces a more powerful effect. It is also of some importance to be able to predict fairly accurately one's reactions in recurring situations. This is also an opportunity to discover to what extent parents or child are inclined to predict catastrophic outcomes, and if that is the case, to help them to make their predictions more realistic.

Summary

The CBT approach can be used with children who have generalised anxiety symptoms or panic attacks, although the details of the therapeutic techniques vary to some extent. The approach may be used with young children who are having difficulty in going to school, or even refusing school. Unfortunately, it may not be possible to engage older children or younger adolescents and their families in whom there is more established school refusal and a long history of behavioural inhibition. There is often a family history of agoraphobia, which complicates the situation. If it is possible to engage the parents and find a way of treating parents with agoraphobia, the CBT approach can still be helpful. Except in this last group, children seem to find the ideas involved in CBT easy to understand, and often three to five sessions are enough to effect change. Under these circumstances, it is sometimes necessary to help the parents catch up with their child. This is important, as a sharing schema for dealing in an adaptive way with potentially anxiety-provoking situations is very powerful.

It is helpful to prepare the child and family for the future. As they progress through the family lifecycle, there are certain stages where there is increased pressure on the child and the symptoms are likely to recur. This is normal, and they can return to the therapist for some further CBT to deal with the symptoms, or very often they are able to deal with them themselves when they know what to expect. I have seen many children return in two, three or four years at such times. They come only once for confirmation, and then cope well with the strategies they have already learnt.

References

American Psychiatric Association (1987) *Diagnostic and Statistical Manual of Mental Disorders: Third Edition-Revised (DSM-III-R)*, Washington, DC: American Psychiatric Association.

American Psychiatric Association (1994) *Diagnostic and Statistical Manual of Mental Disorders: Fourth Edition (DSM-IV)*, Washington, DC: American Psychiatric Association.

Beck, A.T. (1976) *Cognitive Therapy and the Emotional Disorders*, New York: International Universities Press.

Beck, A.T., Rush, A.J., Shaw, B.F. & Emery, G. (1979) *Cognitive Therapy for Depression*, New York: Guilford Press.

Dong, Q., Young, B. & Ollendick, T.H. (1994) 'Fears in Chinese children and adolescents and their relations to anxiety and depression', *Journal of Child Psychology and Psychiatry*, 35(2), pp.351–63.

Hargreaves, R. (1990) *Mr Men and Little Miss Series*, Manchester: World International.

Hawthorn, K., Salkovskis, P.M., Kirk, J. & Clark, D.M. (1993) *Cognitive Behaviour Therapy for Psychiatric Problems: A Practical Guide*, Oxford: Oxford University Press.

Kagan, J., Reznick, J.S., Snidman, N., Gibbons, J. & Johnson, M.O. (1988) 'Childhood derivatives of inhibition and lack of inhibition to the unfamiliar', *Child Development*, 59, pp.1,580–9.

Ollendick, T.H. (1983) 'Reliability and validity of the Revised Fear Survey Schedule for Children (FSSC/R)', *Behaviour Research and Therapy*, 21, pp.685–92.

Ollendick, T.H., King, N.J. & Frary, R.B. (1989) 'Fears in children and adolescents: Reliability and generalizability across gender, age and nationality', *Behaviour Research and Therapy*, 27(1), pp.19–26.

Ollendick, T.H., Yule, W. & Ollier, K. (1991) 'Fears in British children and their relationship to manifest anxiety and depression', *Journal of Child Psychology and Psychiatry*, 32(2), pp.321–31.

Spence, S.H. & McCathie, M. (1993) 'The stability of fears in children: A two years prospective study', *Journal of Child Psychology and Psychiatry*, 34(4), pp.579–85.

Stevenson, J., Batten, N. & Cherner, M. (1992) 'Fears and fearfulness in children and adolescents: A genetic analysis of twin data', *Journal of Child Psychology and Psychiatry*, 33(6), pp.977–85.

Stevenson-Hinde, J. & Shouldice, A. (1995) '4, 5 to 7 years, fearful behaviour, fears and worries', *Journal of Child Psychology and Psychiatry*, 36(6), pp.1,027–38.

Thapar, A. & McGuffin, P. (1995) 'Are anxiety symptoms in childhood heritable?', *Journal of Child Psychology and Psychiatry*, 36(3), pp.439–47.

World Health Organisation (1992) *ICD-10 Classification of Mental and Behavioural Disorders*, Geneva: World Health Organisation.

8 Family therapy

Alec Clark

The childhood task of getting one's needs met

According to William Glasser (1965, 1984), we are all of us 'hard-wired' to have five basic needs satisfied. If they are not satisfied, then acute anxiety and/or depression must result. The needs he indicates are:

- the need to survive and have physiological needs met;
- the need to belong and feel loved;
- the need for power and competence;
- the need for freedom to move and choose for ourselves;
- the need for fun – learning and playing.

He goes on to suggest that although the primacy of any of these needs may vary with individuals, none of them are guaranteed automatic satisfaction. We all of us have to learn the social behaviour required to gain the co-operation of others in their fulfilment. In effect, when we enter the world, we are immediately dependent upon others with whom we have to learn how to negotiate a social contract, and learn the conditions under which they may help (or help us to) satisfy our needs. Usually, some *quid pro quo* is required. Growing babies are expected to coo and gurgle as well as cry, and the first smile is the first down-payment of the returns most parents expect for their investment. Initially, both crying and smiling are pretty spontaneous behaviours, but thereafter, the child will gradually learn how much crying will be rewarded by care and comfort, and how much smiling will turn away wrath.

How families set idiosyncratic conditions

What behaviour by the child elicits what responses from other family members will, of course, depend on the family. All such learning is family- and culturally-specific (see Chapter 13), and children have to learn as they go along. But as each family sets its own conditions under which it will help satisfy a child's needs, and as each family may lay down different conditions for different genders, different ages, or different positions in the family, each child has to embark on quite a steep and unique learning curve, involving a lot of cogitation and experimentation, which, developmentally, may go something like this:

- 'How do I get my needs met in this family?'
- 'How does one get fed around here?'
- 'What do I have to do to get noticed?'
- 'What do you mean, I've got them on the wrong feet?'
- 'You let Susan. Why won't you let me?'
- 'Is "belly" rude?'
- 'What's a period?'
- 'Why do you treat me like a child?'

The growing child is not a passive recipient of experience. She or he is constantly reaching out to make sense of and find meaning in those experiences, and as we shall see later, the search for meaning is a fundamental mechanism for dealing with anxiety.

Anxiety, 'anticipatory anxiety' and normal development

The anxiety provoked when meaning is unclear, or misunderstood, is well illustrated by the instance quoted by Selma Fraiberg (1968, p.122), in which a 2-year-old boy, David, suffered acute anxiety on being told he and his family were to fly to Europe, because he 'didn't know how to fly yet'. Flapping his arms to get airborne was a skill he assumed he would need to acquire in order not to be left behind.

To this understanding must be added the realisation that healthy parenting involves a certain necessary mismatch between a child's needs and desires, and parental willingness to accede to them (McIntee, 1992), leading to some disappointment and anxiety. Without some such mismatch, the child cannot learn how to delay gratification of desires, how to take turns, how to develop new skills. So learning involves a series of small disappointments and transient anxieties. The art is to try to ensure that these are within the child's ability to cope (which coping with disappointment and anxiety is itself a learned skill).

The fact that anxiety is a normal part of the developmental process is further emphasised by Fraiberg (1968, p.11). As children develop, they learn to associate certain events with certain outcomes and to express *anticipatory* anxiety – as a young child might begin to cry or protest as they are taken to their bed in the anticipation of being left alone. Anticipatory anxiety is a necessary and normal physiological and mental preparation for possible danger. It gives the child time to formulate defensive strategies, and to make sense of their experience. It is allied to what Caplan called 'worry work' (1969).

So anxiety cannot and should not be eliminated from childhood experience. It is a natural accompaniment to all novel experiences, and it is that which prompts the child in the search for meaning. It is arguable that if children were not even slightly disturbed by life events, they would cease to be curious, cease to search for answers or work out solutions.

The importance of meaning

Anxiety can therefore be thought of as occupying the gap between experience and learning a meaning. (The child is looking for *a* meaning, not necessarily *the* meaning. All our learning is provisional.) The idea of 'optimum anxiety' has been discussed elsewhere in this volume, but in so far as it is a physiological state triggered by the apprehension of possible danger or challenge, but whose threat has not yet been evaluated (so that the 'fight/flight' dilemma has not yet been resolved), then 'What does this experience mean?' is a burning and urgent question. Only when that question has been answered can the child learn how to behave appropriately. So, if thunder is 'only God moving his furniture around', that 'meaning' may suffice to allay fears in a thunderstorm for the time being. But it is to their carers – the family – that the child must initially turn for such an ascription of meaning, for there is no one else. A parent who says, 'I tell her I'll have her put away if she goes on like that, but she knows I don't mean it', couldn't be more wrong.

The importance of consistency and coherence

It follows that if carers attach inconsistent or contradictory 'meanings' to a child's experience, that child will not know how to prepare for events, organise appropriate behaviour, or construct a coherent story about their lives (Dowling, 1993). This is illustrated by the story of a boy in a children's home, who was always keen to know which carer would be on duty during the night – would it be Sarah or Margaret? Why was it so important to know? Eventually, he confided: 'If I want to go for a wee in the night, Sarah tells me off if I flush the loo because it wakes the others. If it's Margaret, she tells me off if I don't flush it, because it's dirty to leave it. So I need to know.' At first sight, this is an example of a child dealing successfully with inconsistency, but this was *predictable* inconsistency: he knew what to expect from each carer. If Sarah and Margaret had themselves been random, yet demanding, about their 'loo rules', there would have been considerable anxiety, and a few wet beds!

The modern phenomenon of increased family instability, including lack of permanence of caregivers, is clearly an added source of anxiety and worry in this context. There is increasing evidence that even children who appear to have dealt with such disturbing life events as family break-up and the consequent changes in caregiving arrangements may have simply deferred the expression, or even the experience, of that anxiety until later in life (Wallerstein & Blakesee, 1990).

The drive for meaning is so basic that in the absence of adult reassurance about the significance of an event or experience, or in the context of ambivalent or inconsistent adult 'explanations', children are likely to resolve their anxiety by adopting a meaning which may itself be detrimental. If a child is bewildered by life events, or physical pain or assault, they may decide they are utterly helpless, and thus become withdrawn or passive, or (rather) find comfort in the thought that they deserved or caused it in some way. This solution, although provoking its own (secondary) anxiety ('If I caused it, how do I stop it?'), is one way of 'digesting' experience, and it may be preferable to the alternative idea that this environment is hostile to me, or my parents do not love me, and I have no power to change it. In other words, a child will tend to prefer the idea of being a cause to the idea of being a helpless victim.

The child's need for a measure of potency

This 'need to be able to cause' (or to believe what I do can make a difference) satisfies one of our basic needs, the need for potency, mentioned above (Glasser, 1965, 1984). If their sense of belonging and being loved (another basic need) is threatened, then children are not likely to give up their sense of potency and agency as well. But this need to feel instrumental is a potential source of anxiety for a child within a family, especially where other relationships are stressed. So it is a common experience among family workers to find children who have burdened themselves (or who have accepted the burden imposed by others) with the responsibility for family difficulties, and suffer the concomitant anxiety this engenders. Vogel and Savva (1993) suggest the development of an *'Atlas personality'* in adult life of those who, as children, took on adult responsibilities, and were anxious, depressed and crushed by the assumption of a role that was clearly beyond their abilities (see also the story of Kate, pp.132–3).

By the same token, children develop a very strong sense as to whether the family they are in is a safe place in which to divulge or share their anxieties. In abusive or dismissive families, children may learn that any disclosure of distress would itself threaten their security. In such cases, children will attempt to dissemble or defer the direct expression of their anxiety. Thus the young sister of a girl who alleged her father was abusing her consistently denied any of her own abuse over a period of two years, until it became clear that her parents were going to separate anyway. Only then did she also disclose. Her rationale was that she had believed she could save her parents' marriage by keeping quiet. Children will suffer a great deal in order to maintain the illusion of safety and control. In a house of cards, it is better not to breathe a word!

Myth, story and family culture as a source of 'anxiety by proxy'

All families have stories or anecdotes which are designed to imply the need for obedience to certain rules, and the dire consequences of disobedience. In my family, it was: 'Uncle Jack wouldn't eat his greens, and look what happened to him.' When we children asked, 'What did happen to him?', the reply was always, 'Never you mind . . .' I don't think we ever did find out, but it seemed safer to eat our greens, just in case.

Often, the story is hidden – a sort of skeleton in the closet. One of my clients has a mother who is anorexic. Mother is in her sixties now, but is only just telling how *her* mother (my client's deceased grandmother) warned her, when she was a budding adolescent, not to let her brothers notice her developing breasts: 'If they do, they'll tease you unmercifully, as mine did me.' Apparently, mother resolved not to give them a chance. She started dieting heavily, and was still suffering from intermittent amenorrhoea during the early years of her marriage. Mother has continued to 'suffer in silence' ever since (until now) – picking at her food and worrying her family. This last is my point. My client has chronic anxiety problems, having lived with, and still in the shadow of, a mother who always seems to hover on the point of death, but around whom and whose condition a strict taboo is woven. 'Never you mind' can be a powerful engine for anxiety.

A literary example of this anxiety by proxy is the character, Judith Starkadder, in *Cold Comfort Farm* (Gibbons, 1932). It is Aunt Ada Doom who 'saw something nasty in the woodshed', but it is the next generation, especially her niece, Judith, which shows all the signs of carrying the burden of that experience, without ever knowing what it was. ('Never you mind'!)

Evidence has also accumulated on the second-generation effect of the Holocaust. Parker (1983) has emphasised the role of excessive parental anxiety in overprotective parenting, and Halik et al. (1990) have commented that Holocaust survivors are often handicapped in helping their children deal with separation anxiety and individuation, because separation from their own parents was often abrupt, brutal, and never fully resolved.

The basis for a family approach

The argument for a family approach in the treatment of childhood anxiety is thus very strong. Not only does such an approach help the therapist to make a more global assessment, thus decreasing the risk of pathologising the child, it also helps other family members to acknowledge the 'worry work' the child may be doing on their behalf, and to be appraised of the significance of their own behaviours and expectations, and provides them the opportunity to give appropriate assurances to the child. This approach can also unmask relevant myths and family stories, as mentioned above.

The family approach is useful in helping parents deal with some of the normal transitional experiences, like the arrival of a sibling, and the normal developmental landmarks, but I believe it is *vital* where a child is showing stress in the following cases:

- death or loss in the family;
- changes and/or inconsistencies in caregiving;
- the division of loyalties implicit in a split family.

In the context of abuse or fear of abuse, family therapy is not indicated, as this is the last place a child will choose to share such fears. But in the post-disclosure period, when family members are needing to regroup around the acknowledged trauma, then again I regard the family approach as highly desirable.

Examples of family work with childhood anxiety

Not all the following examples are equally 'weighty', but they do illustrate the variety of techniques available within the family therapy approach, including the use of strategy (Haley, 1986), 'externalising the problem' and the use of letter-writing (White & Epstein, 1989), 'sculpting' or family modelling (Simon, 1972) and 'parts work', a therapy model developed by David Calof of the Family Psychotherapy Practice, Seattle.

Simon: A case of 'developmental anxiety'

I met Simon (aged 4) and his sister, Sarah (aged 6), only once, together with their parents. Although he was doing well at his new school, he was becoming increasingly clingy and demanding at home, seeming to need help with skills he had already achieved, and needing company late into the night and whenever he went to the toilet. My first reaction was to encourage his parents to praise his school achievements and to give clear approval every time he achieved a developmental milestone – perhaps using Sarah as someone he could measure himself against.

But on reflection, after the session, I realised that Simon needed to have more control over how grown-up he was, so I wrote the following message to the parents:

> Instead of challenging him (even by implication) that he is getting too big to have you do for him things he can manage by himself at school, I suggest you both take the initiative and offer to do various things for him or with him until he tells you he is ready to do these things by himself.
>
> I suggest you tell him, 'If you want to go to the toilet, come and tell one of us and we will come with you unless you tell us you want to go by yourself. When it is time to dress or undress, one of us will offer to do it, unless you tell us you want to try by yourself. One of us will cut your meat, unless and until you tell us you would like to have a go yourself.' Assume he needs you, until he tells you otherwise.

The parents wrote back, telling of a real change. A struggle for dependence began to transform into a struggle for independence, and 'I can't – you help me' was transformed into 'I can do it!' Strategic techniques have been criticised as being disrespectful – perhaps fooling a family or an individual into attaining a desired goal by telling them not to (Whan, 1983), but I believe the strategy outlined above respected both the parents' wishes and the boy's needs.

A mother and daughter face the aftermath of sexual abuse

When I met Janis, she was 13. Her father had been convicted of sexually abusing her, and was in custody. Her mother shared in the session. Not only was Janis carrying the burden of her own abuse; she was also carrying guilt and anxiety over the break-up of the family, and what seemed to be ambivalent signals from mother about who had been to blame.

White and Epston (1989) show the advantage of treating family problems as 'external' to those who are carrying them, and in my own work, I have sometimes taken this notion quite literally. In this case, I gave Janis a chair to carry, and suggested that the chair could represent all kinds of guilt and anxiety that she was carrying. I speculated with mother as to who could give her daughter permission to put the chair down. At first, mother insisted that only father could do that, and that he was neither available nor willing. However, as Janis began to struggle with the weight of the chair, mother began to realise the significance of her own position, and she was able to say very gently, 'Janis, you don't need to carry that for me ...'

White and Epston also point to the merit of using letters to confirm newly-recognised relationships and responsibilities, so, in recognition of what her daughter needed to hear from her, and what she needed to say, mother composed the following letter in the session and gave it to her daughter:

> Dear Janis
>
> I want you to know that because of what happened between you and your dad, I have been through hell.
>
> This has made it very difficult for me to think clearly, and sometimes I have felt very angry with you, as well as with your dad.
>
> But I now want you to know that I love you very much, and hold you in no way responsible for what happened, and I bear you no grudge.
>
> Love Mum xxx

Janis asked her mother to spell out what 'bearing no grudge' meant. She then hugged her mother with tears in her eyes.

'Putting worries in the bin': A case of school phobia

Kate, aged 10, was the middle of three children of a middle-class family which seemed to have been facing a series of unconnected disasters when I met them. Father had been made redundant, and their house had been repossessed; mother had undergone hospitalisation and a hysterectomy; one grandfather (a favourite) had been committed for psychiatric treatment (and granny had commented that Kate would end up the same way, she worried so much!), and the other grandmother was terminally ill.

In the midst of all this, Kate had developed intense anxiety about attending school. She had also begun to have difficulty eating, fearing that something might get stuck in her throat. However, when I met her, together with her 4-year-old brother, her 14-year-old sister and her parents, she had already begun to deal with some of her phobias, although she had not attended school consistently for the last three months.

During the first session, she elected to show me her 'red book' – a sort of secret diary in bold red ballpoint. In it, she had recorded some of her fears, including her fear of choking, but also a fear that mummy and daddy might split up. She confided that the choking wasn't a problem any more, because she had just told herself it was silly. But she was very worried about mummy and daddy.

Her parents and her sister sought to reassure her, but to little avail. In order to discover what role she was perceived as playing in her family, I suggested a sculpt (Simon, 1972), which was conducted by her sister, Susan. Susan placed Kate on mother's knee, and sat father next to mother, with his arm round mother's shoulder. Father's hand was thus just next to Kate's head as she sat on her mother's knee. I suggested to Kate that she notice this, and asked her who or what she thought was keeping dad's arm round mum. She replied: 'Me!'

Diagnostically, this was quite significant. As I noted above, children often feel they have a role in keeping the family together, and here was a child making that belief quite explicit. It is also interesting to note how family myths (e.g. the link granny was making between mental illness and worry) played their part and intensified Kate's symptoms. I intervened as follows:

1 I encouraged both parents to thank Kate for her concern.
2 I encouraged them to offer Kate some 'worry time', when she could relieve herself of some of her worries with one or both of them (perhaps bedtime), and to make a clear distinction between her need to worry and her need to go to school.
3 I suggested that the least 'fraught' parent should be the one to help Kate to get to school. Father was chosen. (To my mind, speculation about the possible shift in family dynamics implied in this solution is academic. I do not believe that successful therapy needs a theory of pathology.)

After a few sessions, Kate was going to school unaided, and proudly announced: 'I've shoved my worries in the bin.' Following White and Epston (1989), to celebrate her victory, I awarded her the following certificate:

Victory over Worries
Certificate
This certificate is awarded to . . . .
for shoving her worries in the bin,
and not letting them get the better of her.
If anyone wants to know how she did it,
she will be pleased to tell them.
Awarded on the . . . . day of . . . .
Signed . . . .

'How little is little?': A boy overcomes his fear of being left alone

I met Mark when he was 8, together with his 10-year-old sister, Ruth, and their parents. After watching a TV film about a child being left alone, he had become extremely phobic about being left alone, and would hardly let his mother out of his sight. This included following her to the toilet, and waiting inside school at the end of each day until his sister could inform him that mother had arrived in the car. The children lived only a few minutes' walk away from school. Father volunteered that he had been a very nervous child, and that he therefore knew how Mark felt.

My general line with fear and phobias is to try to help children find a way of being relatively comfortable with uncomfortable feelings. One way of doing this is to employ what David Calof calls 'parts work'. He makes the assumption that 'parts' of our personalities carry (say) fear, or other emotions – possibly on behalf of other family members – and that other 'parts' may either be critical ('I'm just being silly') or may be able to offer a more mature and helpful attitude to the felt problem. In other words, the solution is in the client, not in the therapist.

I decided to use this approach in this case, and therefore took the following steps:

1   I asked Mark if he was willing to experience a bit of his anxiety about where mother was, in the room, so that we could all appreciate what it was like for him, and see how he coped with it. He gave his permission.
2   I sat him with his face to the wall, so that he couldn't see any other family members, and told him that in a moment he would hear the door open and close, and that it was possible that this was his mother leaving the room. But he wouldn't know, as he couldn't see.
3   I signalled to other family members to stay where they were, opened and closed the office door, then took a seat beside Mark.
4   The following conversation took place (for some reason, this whole conversation was conducted in a whisper. This was not my conscious intention, but it seemed to produce a hypnotic, conspiratorial effect on both of us. See O'Hanlon and Martin, 1992.):

> *Th*: Where's mother now?
> *M*: I don't know.
> *Th*: What's it like, not knowing?
> *M*: It makes me feel a bit panicky.
> *Th*: What do you feel like doing?
> *M*: I feel like turning round, to see if she's there . . .

Th: A bit scary.

M: Yes.

Th: So, the scared part of Mark could get very panicky, and want to turn round. You can feel that now, yes?

M: Yes.

Th: So I'm just sitting here wondering how Mark is coping with all those feelings, yet he isn't turning round. He isn't checking out. Can you explain that to me?

M: Well, I think there's a part of me saying it's alright.

Th: You mean, as well as a little-boy Mark that feels scared, there is also another part, like a big boy, that is saying, 'It's alright, I'll look after you'?

M: That's right. Yes.

Th: So you can feel both parts – the little-boy part, and the big-boy part?

M: Yes.

Th: That's wonderful . . . I wonder if you can do something even more . . . I wonder if you can now imagine yourself in a panicky place –

M: At school –

Th: What's happening?

M: The car hasn't come –

Th: Oh, and that makes little Mark scary, yes?

M: Yes.

Th: And what about big Mark. Is he there?

M: He could be.

Th: If he was there, what would he do? Can you imagine him there?

M: Yes. I think he would say, 'It's alright. She'll come soon.'

Th: That's wonderful. Tell me more about big Mark. Tell me, does big Mark know the way home – the way to walk home?

M: Yes.

Th: Just check that out. Imagine you are big Mark, and you are setting out to walk home from school – with Ruth, perhaps. Just keep your eyes closed and imagine that walk home, just to see if there are any snags – pavements – streets – trees . . . (pause) . . . would that be alright?

M: Yes. I could do that.

Th: Well, I want to congratulate big Mark for looking after little Mark so well. Would you like to turn round now?

Mark turned round, and after a little while, he and his sister were able to negotiate what days of the week they would find their own way home from school, rather than being met by the car. In doing so, they also had to overcome their mother's anxiety!

A month later, mother reported that Mark preferred not to be met, and that although he still 'tried it on', if parents wanted to go out at night, leaving the children with grandparents, all in all, the situation had improved.

Comment

The cases I have chosen reflect my growing interest in 'solution-focused' therapy in the midst of a general family therapy modality (George et al., 1990). In other words, although I try to stay aware of what may be the deeper family structures which may be maintaining anxiety for a particular child, I usually aim to help the child deal with those anxieties, without necessarily attending to their source. This was clearly the case in the last example, in which I decided not to explore the father's admission that he, too, suffered anxiety as a child.

In some cases, it may seem that I am therefore offering child-centred therapy in the presence of the family, rather than thorough-going systemic therapy (where relationships past and present are *the* focus of the work). However, I also subscribe to the view that even if other family members seem to be merely witnesses to the therapeutic process, the effect on them and their relationships will not be insignificant. All the approaches in this chapter are offered on the implicit or explicit assumption that others besides the child will need to change if therapy is to be successful. In that sense, family therapy and/or systemic theory should not be viewed as disparate alternatives to other approaches suggested elsewhere, but as one of the dimensions to be considered, whatever approach is being used.

References

Caplan, G. (1969) *An Approach to Community Mental Health*, London: Tavistock Publications.

Dowling, E. (1993) 'Are family therapists listening to the young?', *Journal of Family Therapy*, 15(4), pp.403–11.

Fraiberg, S.H. (1968) *The Magic Years*, London: Methuen.

George, E., Iveson, C. & Ratner, H. (1990) *Problem to Solution: Brief Therapy with Individuals and Families*, London: Brief Therapy Press.

Gibbons, S. (1932) *Cold Comfort Farm*, London: Allen Lane.

Glasser, W. (1965) *Reality Therapy*, New York: Harper & Row.

Glasser, W. (1984) *Control Theory*, New York: Harper & Row.

Haley, J. (1986) *Uncommon Therapy*, London and New York: W.W. Norton.

Halik, V., Rosenthal, D.A. & Pattison, E. (1990) 'Intergenerational effects of the Holocaust: Patterns of engagement in the mother–daughter relationship', *Family Process*, 29(3), pp.325–39.

McIntee, J. (1992) *Trauma: The Psychological Process*, Chester: The Chester Therapy Centre.

O'Hanlon, W.H. & Martin, M. (1992) *Solution Oriented Hypnosis*, London and New York: W.W. Norton.

Parker, G. (1983) *Parental Overprotection: Risk Factors in Psychosocial Development*, New York: Grune and Stratton.

Simon, R. (1972) 'Sculpting the family', *Family Process*, 11(1), pp.49–57.
Vogel, L.Z. & Savva, S. (1993) 'Atlas personality', *British Journal of Medical Psychology*, 66, pp.323–30.
Wallerstein, J. & Blakesee, S. (1990) *Second Chances*, London: Bantam.
Whan, M. (1983) 'Tricks of the trade: Questionable theory and practice in family therapy', *British Journal of Social Work*, 13(3), pp.321–37.
White, M. & Epston, D. (1989) *Literate Means to Therapeutic Ends*, Australia: Dulwich Centre Publications.

9 Play therapy

Mary Gray

Play Therapy is the dynamic process between child and Play Therapist, in which the child explores, at his or her own pace and with his or her own agenda, those issues past and current, conscious and unconscious, that are affecting the child's life in the present. The child's inner resources are enabled by the therapeutic alliance to bring about growth and change. Play Therapy is child centred, in which play is the primary medium and speech is the secondary medium. (Association of Play Therapists, 1995, p.1)

Historically, play therapy was begun in the 1930s and 1940s by Anna Freud, Melanie Klein, Donald Winnicott and Margaret Lowenfeld (Cattanach, 1992). Freud founded the Hampstead War Nurseries, which was later to become the Anna Freud Centre for Psychoanalytic Study and Treatment of Children. Before starting the therapy, the children lived in an atmosphere of love and caring which they could really depend upon. By observing their play, she felt that children's problems were replayed – their real-life events and the exploration of the world they live in. Close observation was the key. What struck the worker about the child's play was recorded immediately. This is an integral part of training today.

Winnicott observed children's preoccupation with playing as parallel with adults' concentration in the real world. Winnicott recognised the importance of the relationship between mother and child while they played creatively. The transitional object (security blanket, soft toy) which represents the mother acts as a defence against the anxiety of separation. Therefore, play is the infant's way of coping with emotions, excitement, anxiety and fear, through the interpretation of play, a bridging of the gap between inner experiences and the reality of the outside world.

Lowenfeld (1950), a children's physician, became interested in the psychological aspects of children's illness. Through play, she made direct contact with the thoughts, feelings and desires of children, with herself as the interested adult in the role of a playmate. The 'world' technique (which involves the use of a sandtray, into which are added toys, other objects and sometimes water, with which the child can create a picture) was the principal tool which helped children to 'say' what they wanted and allowed them to think entirely in a non-verbal manner. This language has to be learned by the therapist as the child tries to make sense of the world around themself, their experiences and their reaction to them, which, through the 'world' technique, can be unravelled, sorted and integrated.

Klein believed it was necessary to have a carefully-designed playroom. She believed that play was like an adult's free association, and it needed profound interpretation, as it revealed unconscious anxieties and fantasies. The feelings the child aroused in the therapist may have been the child's own feelings projected onto the therapist, and the relationship between the child and the therapist was similar to the early mother–child experience. Unconscious conflicts were believed by Klein and Freud to be the source of many childhood psychiatric disorders, and bringing the unconscious elements to consciousness would help in the resolution of the anxiety and the strengthening of the child's ego.

Play therapy is usually conducted in a specially-adapted playroom equipped with play materials such as doll's houses, castles, puppet theatres, sandtrays, dressing-up boxes, etc. These play materials can function as psychological containers. The child selects the container which could become the background for the stories about their lives. This can be something which has happened to them personally, or something which has happened to others which they were witness to; all of which, when explored, widens and deepens the child's story and leads them to find their own personal resolution.

In the playroom that I use, the toys are kept in large bags with drawstring tops, and thus the toys can be selected carefully or tipped out, one bag at a time. Each bag contains different types of toys. One has a doll's house, people and furniture; another is a 'scary' bag, with wild and domestic animals and fantasy figures; a third contains hero and villain figures, inspired by the media at the present time; a fourth is a 'transport' bag with vehicles, roads, fences, grass, trees and houses; another is a puppet bag, with family members – mothers and fathers, sisters and brothers, kings, queens, witches and wizards, animal families, and animals from fairy stories, like wolves, for example. A special bag contains toys that offer sound, sight and touch experiences. Finally, the usual arts and crafts materials are available.

There are two methods of play therapy; the differences between them lie in the interaction between the therapist and the child. The first is child-centred play therapy, and is based on the fact that play is the child's natural medium of self-expression, and the theory that the child has an ability to solve their own problems satisfactorily. The therapist provides the play setting within safe boundaries which make this healing play possible, offering the child a containing relationship and a mental space in which the child's anxieties can be expressed and thought about. Alertness and reflective listening are the therapist's most powerful tools. They offer the child insight into their own experiences, attitudes, thoughts and feelings, allowing for growth, maturity and fulfilment.

The second method, focused play therapy, is helpful in saving time and shortening therapy, as well as making sure that vital areas of assessment and therapy are covered (Oaklander, 1978). The task is to help children feel strong inside and to see the world around them as it really is, to know that they have choices, and to give them the strength to make those choices.

Play therapists need a language to use with adults to bridge the gap between a child's experience and the adult's need to understand. Specific techniques help the child to express their feelings. Stories are developed in which the child employs the use of symbols and metaphors. Jung (according to Grainger, 1990) defines symbols as images and emotions that gain psychic energy. Metaphors work in the right-hand hemisphere of the brain by means of communicating with both the conscious and unconscious mind simultaneously. While the conscious mind tells the story in concepts, ideas, stories and images, the unconscious mind is slipped the therapeutic messages which evoke new behavioural responses. Therapeutic suggestions are integrated in stories, jokes and anecdotes.

Robert, a 12-year-old boy, was abandoned by his mother and stepfather when they returned to another country, and he lived with his grandmother. He used symbols from the game of football to describe his pain. Robert and his siblings were the winning team, his parents were footballs which could be kicked around, and his grandmother was the red card which had the power to send players off the field. When the playdough shapes were mixed together, they became dinosaurs: a strong carnivore and a weak herbivore. Robert's dinosaurs became Rob and Bert, who were imprisoned and separated from each other in different cells. The strong one had to rescue the weak one before they both died; instead, they both escaped by running away. Robert had been persistently running away, placing himself in great danger. It appeared that in his weak moments, triggers from his past life-experiences made him take flight, and he would commit minimal offences which brought out his fearless responses.

Play therapy is helpful in identifying what has been a much too painful event to live with and understand. The therapist watches to see if the child knows what to do with toys, and may need to encourage the child to be able to 'play'. When the child begins to handle the toys, the therapist should notice how the child handles them, which toys become important, which toys are avoided. Is the energy of the child's play frantic, pathetic or hesitant?

Rebecca was 6 years old, and lived in a family where she constantly witnessed violence towards her mother by her stepfather. She felt unable to even peek into the 'scary' toy bag. As it was possible that she might need a toy from it for her future play therapy sessions, she asked me to take them out one at a time while she watched from the other side of the room. Whenever Rebecca needed one of the toys from this bag, she would ask me to get it for her.

Anxiety and play therapy

Play is held to be 'cathartic'. The discharge of emotions through play in a safe environment can reduce the child's anxiety. The child is given 'permission' to act out conflicts and unacceptable impulses, after which the child will have the ability to adjust more easily to normal social demands.

Sigmund Freud (1955) described psychic trauma as an injury to the personality which happens as a result of anxiety so sudden, intense and unexpected that it overwhelms ordinary coping and defensive mechanisms.

Terr (1990), who observed children's play for several years after they had been kidnapped, suggests 11 characteristics of post-traumatic play which distinguish it from ordinary play:

- compulsive repetition;
- unconscious link between the play and the traumatic event;
- literalness of play, with simple defences only;
- failure to relieve anxiety;
- wide age range;
- varying time lag prior to its development;
- conveying power to non-traumatised youngsters;
- contagion to new generations of children;
- danger;
- use of doodling, talking, typing and audio duplications in modes of repeated play;
- the possibility of therapeutically retracing post-traumatic play to an earlier trauma. (Terr, 1983, p.309)

Children who come to my playroom have been referred either because of their behaviour or because of the anxiety of the professionals who have responsibility for them. The children exhibit many of the characteristics seen by Terr.

Mary, aged 6, played out dramatically her experience of being taken into fostercare because her mother was admitted into hospital for detoxification. As the weeks progressed, there was a compulsive repetition of the entire play sequence, with Mary taking on each of the roles of the child, mother, nurse, fosterparent and social worker. Mary ended the play suddenly by announcing that she didn't want to play this sequence any more.

Anna was 13 months old when she was weaned from the breast. The process was difficult for both child and mother, because breastfeeding had been a satisfying experience for them both. Anna then developed a bladder infection and was catheterised. Anna's mother responded to her distress by offering the breast, and both were comforted by this. Breastfeeding continued until Anna was 2, when she was once more weaned. The subsequent play indicated a time lag between the original traumatic event, in this case the catheterisation, and the post-traumatic play. Anna played in a nurturing way with her doll. However, when changing the doll's nappy, she tore out the legs and threw them across the room. This play re-enactment occurred over a period of two months. At the same time, Anna played with a cow and calf, which was torn from the udders when feeding and thrown across the room. Anna was offered the opportunity to be the doctor and the mother, as I verbally acknowledged both the doll's and the calf's feelings, and the play began to normalise to a nurturing nappy change and a verbal acknowledgement of the calf's feelings.

During his assessment period, Tony, a 10-year-old boy who had set a fire in a factory and caused several thousand pounds' worth of damage to a building site, built an elaborate sandtray story. The sand was divided through the middle, with cars neatly lined up one side; on the other were rows of wild animals. The instamatic camera had run out of film, and I had to go into the cupboard to replace it. When I was ready to take the photo, Tony stood with his hands fidgeting in his pocket, the sandtray was empty and the sand was smoothed over. This showed that the good and bad sides of Tony were too difficult to endure, and this play had failed to relieve him of his anxiety.

Terry, a 3-year-old boy, had witnessed violence between his parents when his father had tried to strangle his mother. When Terry played, he began to tie long strips of paper around the necks of dolls and his play friends. In the nursery he attended, Terry's play caused distress as he communicated and enacted episodes with children who had not experienced this trauma. After being given the safe setting of play therapy and the opportunity to play, Terry's play in the nursery normalised.

Peter, a 6-year-old boy who had been excluded from his primary school, was excited to have a photo taken of his sandtray story, which we packed away while the photo was developing. When he looked at the photo, two or three minutes later, its effect caused such an anxiety attack that he rushed under the table and curled up into a ball, rocking to and fro to express the fear he was experiencing. In this instance, the play process had become as dangerous to the child as the event itself.

Daniel was a 10-year-old boy whose mother said he was being naughty at home and in school. At the first session, while playing Winnicott's scribble drawing, he casually wrote 'help' on the paper. The theme continued through every story for 12 weeks, until he was able to feel safe enough to say that access to his father was so frightening that he did not wish to go any more. His greatest fear was that his father would fail to return him to his mother.

The children described thus far have illustrated particular issues encountered in the play therapy process. The following case examples of Andrew, aged 6, and Penny, aged 11, will illustrate the stages a child can be enabled to experience and the interaction that takes place within the contract developed with that child.

Andrew

Andrew was referred at the point of being excluded from his second school. His mother feared he would become a psychopath, and could find nothing positive to say about her son. Andrew's father had committed suicide, having taken an overdose the previous year. The school found Andrew very difficult to control. He was reported to be always in the middle of any disturbances or fighting that happened in both classroom and playground. He also had poor concentration span, which was having an effect on his educational progress. Although the grounds for Andrew's referral appeared at first to be antisocial behaviour, it soon became apparent that the presenting problem was actually covert fear and anxiety.

There had been no mention of Andrew having a sleep disturbance, yet by the third session a theme was emerging, and I felt it was important to ask Andrew's mother about his sleeping pattern. It proved to be the case that he was having problems with sleeping, which she viewed as more 'naughty' behaviour.

Andrew was the eldest of two children. His sister, Emily, two years younger, presented as a perfect child. Andrew's parents had separated before his father, Lawrence, committed suicide, but Andrew still had contact with his paternal grandparents. Dean was Andrew's mother's boyfriend. Andrew referred to him as 'Dean' or 'my new dad'. Throughout the period of therapy, he was confused about Dean's role.

At the beginning of the first session, Andrew was quiet, looking through a toy bag and handing each toy to me when he had played with it. He eventually played with the toys with an element of surprise in them. For example, as Andrew slowly took the lid off an exploding tin, he smiled at me as the tension mounted. Then together we laughed at my response when I physically jumped. Andrew did the same with the pop-up ghost, adding ghostly/spooky noises to it. Then Andrew indicated that it was my turn to do the same to him. This turn-taking continued for a time, and Andrew began to share information about his friends at school, bigger boys who would start trouble in which he was always involved. He proudly told me that there was one friend who was smaller than him whom he could catch, and when he did, he would always batter him.

At the second appointment, Andrew chose to play with the sandtray, and he set out a scene from his house: everyone was asleep in bed. Suddenly, he was woken up by the noise of Dean being sick from having drunk too much beer (Andrew had used a Razblaster, a toy with a long balloon tongue which reaches down into a toilet and makes a raspberry noise when it is squeezed). Andrew watched Dean being sick on the carpet and then returned to his bed. Andrew took the small doll boy representing himself and put it into bed. However, he could not sleep, and using a small popgun, he shot Dean.

At the third session, Andrew made playdough shapes with small pastry-cutting shapes to symbolise each family member. These dough shapes, when put together, became a Tyrannosaurus Rex. The T. Rex was playing in the jungle, fighting with his dinosaur friends. Upstairs in his bedroom were toys that he wanted to play with, but it was too frightening for the T. Rex to get them. He needed his mother's help, because there was a ghost in his wardrobe and she could frighten it away. (During this week, Andrew had been to see the movie *Jurassic Park*, which is recommended for 12 years and upwards.)

As Andrew left the playroom, he expressed his desire to play with the 'shaky pen' in the next session. When he entered the playroom for his fourth session, he went straight to, and picked up, the shaky pen and proceeded to draw a frightened family: Dean (mother's boyfriend), mum, Andrew and Emily (his sister). They were attacked by a horrible ghost who lived in the next town. He had burgled the family home, the punishment for which was death, where you became all bones. Andrew's natural father came from this town, and was still living there when he took his own life. Andrew asked me what happened to people when they die. I told him I was not really sure, and asked him what he thought happened. He said they became all bones, because the worms ate them.

As Andrew's theme throughout the four sessions had the physical element of fighting, I suggested to Andrew at his fifth session that it might be fun to play in the padded soft-cushion room. This was to allow Andrew the opportunity to express himself in the physical coping strategy he naturally used in his life, in a caring environment where he would find acceptance and also be physically safe.

I introduced 'The Balloon Game', an exercise which can deal with loss and/or separation. It is a very physical game, and it enabled Andrew to throw himself around in a padded-cushion room. By the end of the session, he was very tired, hot and out of breath. During this session, he was very aggressive in his play, wanting to burst his own balloon. It is very unusual to observe a child not wanting to protect their own balloon in this game.

Following this session, in which Andrew had displayed aggression, I felt it would be useful for him to continue this theme, and suggested that maybe he could use clay, because clay, no matter how hard it is played with in a destructive manner, can be returned to its original shape. Andrew enjoyed the clay, punching, pinching and throwing it. He was feeling angry with his mum, as she and Dean were going on holiday without him and his sister. With the clay, he made two strong men (himself and Dean), who sailed away to the island of Tenerife. They were attacked by a shark, and drowned. Their bodies were washed up on the beach, where rescue services brought them back to life. Andrew said he believed that if he was a strong man, then he would not die, he could come back to life – in fact, he could live forever.

Andrew was curious in this session about the other naughty boys who played with me. He thought he knew a boy in his class who must come and play with me too. To boost Andrew's self-esteem, I expressed my surprise, and acknowledged his thoughts that I played with naughty boys. I explained that lots of grown-ups see some behaviour as naughty, but I felt this was a way children tried to express their feelings of sadness, anger or fear, and it sometimes comes out in a way that it is difficult to understand, so grown-ups call it 'naughty'. Andrew then said: 'I'm sad. My real dad died, you know.'

At the seventh session, Andrew arrived, announcing that he would like to do a puppet show. The main parts were Batman and Robin fighting the Joker, who wanted to kill Lawrence. 'That's my real dad's name,' Andrew announced. The Joker was successful, shooting Andrew's dad. Batman and Robin found him too late. They did, however, bury him and put flowers on his grave. When his mother saw Andrew's story the following week, she said that it would soon be Lawrence's anniversary, and they would be visiting his grave. Andrew's mother went on to say that when his father was buried, Andrew had attended the funeral. When the coffin was lowered into the ground, he had tried to jump in to get his dad back, so that the worms wouldn't eat him. Interestingly, mother's response to this was: 'You had to laugh.'

The tenth and eleventh sessions were spent with a sand story, concentrating on a strong man in his bed, who was visited by a ghost at night. Andrew made the ghost from tissue paper stuck to a slime ball, which flashed a red light and made a scary ghost 'whoo' noise. Using slime, Andrew covered the strong man, who was then unable to move, an expression of paralysed fear. Andrew then took the popgun and shot the ghost. During these sessions, Andrew was very quiet and thoughtful, perhaps resolving his fears at a much deeper level. There was a change in Andrew's interaction with me during these two sessions. He had appeared more contained, calmer and thoughtful in his play.

I therefore presented the 'House Tree Person' exercise, in which a piece of paper is folded into four. In the first square, Andrew drew a person who became Elvis Presley. On a recent holiday, mother had been present at a competition for Elvis impressionists. Andrew said 'He was dead, you know,' and continued to draw a skeleton in a coffin under the person. The house was Elvis's house, which was no longer safe without him to look after it, and he drew Elvis's ghost going up the stairs. The walls might fall down, or robbers might come and break into it. Quickly, Andrew drew the tree full of robbers watching and waiting outside Elvis's house. Then Andrew announced that he wanted to draw in the fourth square (some children draw in it, others do not). Andrew drew his family: Dean, new dad (who was about to move in permanently), mum, Emily and himself, announcing: 'This is a happy family who will live for ever and ever.'

Andrew's mother was very pleased with Andrew's progress, and her feelings towards him had begun to change. She now expressed the feeling that she 'liked him sometimes'. Andrew's schoolteacher was equally pleased with his progress academically. He was four weeks ahead of his attainment targets. His teacher reported that within the classroom and in the playground, Andrew's behaviour had changed. He was no longer involved in fighting, and she had observed him moving away from any trouble as it was building. Instead, she noticed that he had begun to comfort those children who had problems or who were in distress.

Penny

Penny and her family were experiencing considerable stress because of the violence between her two teenage brothers, aged 15 and 18 years. Penny, the youngest of five children, suffered from bedwetting at night.

She was also being bullied at school by her peers. Penny's father had left the family three years previously, after 22 years of marriage. At the time of Penny's birth, her father had an accident at work, during which he suffered a head injury. There had been a history of alcohol abuse and violent behaviour towards both his wife and his children, which increased after the accident. The other two daughters, aged 20 and 22 years, no longer lived at home.

When Penny came to the first appointment, she was very shy and quiet. The 'Six Piece Story' exercise enables the therapist to find the child's coping mechanisms in story form. It also allows the child to find solutions to their problems. The main character in Penny's 'Six Piece Story' was a small sunflower, which was crying and in need of some more water to grow. The problem was that other sunflowers would not share the water, and always came before her.

At the second session, using Penny's story, she made sunflowers for a play in order to extend the story, hoping to find a solution for the sunflower. In the interaction between the five sunflowers, it was highlighted that there was one very selfish sunflower. This one needed to be made aware of its behaviour by the other sunflowers and support the main character to get enough water for it to survive. Penny felt it was important to have her needs heard. It was equally important to be able to tell her family about those needs.

At the third session, the family were in crisis, each in their own way acting out. The brothers had been drinking and fighting, while Penny, her sisters and her mother were feeling ill. They expressed that they were very anxious: the anniversary of their father leaving was upon them. Penny's session focused on her father leaving and living near the sea. Penny felt that she did not want to go and see him, but hoped that he would be happy living there.

At the fourth session, with the aid of the 'Button Tree' exercise, Penny was able to explore the different family members' interactions within the family. Penny found it difficult to speak to the button that represented her father, and expressed that one brother had begun to 'act out' like her father. Penny's mother was unable to protect her from her father's and brothers' violence, as she herself was afraid of them. In fact, Penny's mother turned to Penny for support.

For the ninth session, to enable Penny to look at a new beginning when her father left home, I asked her to paint a feeling she felt at the time. At first, she was anxious about the process and couldn't begin. I encouraged her to squiggle a shape, any shape, and this she was able to do. To fill it in, Penny began to spot and blob, which then became flick-painting. As the paint escaped the shape, Penny let out sighs and sounds like anxiety being released. By the end of the session, Penny looked physically more relaxed.

At the tenth session, I asked Penny to paint the feeling of what it felt like to live at home with her dad. This she was unable to do. I then asked Penny to paint what she might have learnt from the experience. Penny painted a field of bulb flowers, with two beautiful roses, to which Penny wrote an equally beautiful response. The two roses, Penny later explained, were her mother and sister, and she revealed that she would like to be a rose like them one day.

Penny's friend was in a crisis this week, as it was the anniversary of her mother leaving the family. Penny became anxious as she spoke, shedding tears while saying how difficult it was for her to listen to her friend's pain, as it evoked all Penny's losses. I reflected that Penny was indeed a rose, too.

At the eleventh session, Penny had no problem painting her feelings of her hope of what the future would be for her. This she expressed with three flowers, with three hearts next to them, symbolising her mother, sister and herself. There was real hope for the future.

I believe that Penny was often expected to support the family during their crises. Penny appeared willing to do this; however, emotionally, she was not equipped to do so. The family situation had now changed, and it became impossible for Penny to continue with her sessions, but she needed reassurance that she could return in the future if it became necessary. Indeed, within a few weeks, Penny's mother contacted me. The expected move had not happened, and Penny was in distress over the death of her 12-year-old dog. She began wetting the bed again, and bullying had started at her new school as a result. To acknowledge the loss of the dog, we did several sessions on an 'Endings Book', which helped Penny to cope. Her doctor prescribed her with a nasal spray to help her with the enuresis, and the bullying problem at school subsided.

The family history during the period I had worked with them showed a pendulum swing from crisis to euphoria, with nothing in between. Before the work on the 'Endings Book' was completed, the elder sister announced plans to marry later on that year, and Penny was to be a bridesmaid. This showed the swing from the dog's death and the deep loss suddenly turning into joy because of being a bridesmaid for the first time. Penny and I discussed these points, and agreed that it would be useful to explore them in the next two sessions.

Penny chose to make a happy/sad doll with clay. The joyful side was dressed in the proposed bridesmaid dress in the colours Penny would like, and the sad side was dressed in old, worn-out clothes. (Incidentally, when the clay dried, it accidentally leaned forward on the sad side, looking downhearted and upward on the smiling side.)

For these two sessions, Penny drew a pie chart and divided up the feelings she experienced. Hysterical/funny was a quarter of the positive side, and fear was a quarter of the shadow side. Penny said that if I lived her life, I would feel fear too.

Penny felt unable to begin the painting, admitting that it was always difficult to begin most pieces of work at school and with me. However, with encouragement, Penny chose the colours she would like for her bridesmaid dress. The colours took shape and became a beautiful flower. The story of the flower was that it was 8 years old when it began to grow outside a beautiful house in the spring and summer, and it was taken into the house as autumn approached, where it was admired by everyone who lived there. Penny was 8 years old when her father left.

At the next session, I asked Penny if it was possible to see a cross-section of the beautiful flower, to see what the plant's beginning looked like. Penny painted a bulb in the soil. This beautiful flower grew from the bulb in a beautiful red pot. It had been picked by a little girl, planted and put in a shed in the dark at the bottom of the garden. Telling the story and then exploring it through the metaphor, Penny became very sad in her body language and facial expression. I felt that this was the piece of work which Penny had avoided in the 'Hello/Goodbye' second stage.

When Penny attended the next session, she had not been to school for three days. Her mother didn't know why or what the matter was. Penny admitted that for two weeks she had become very tired and unable to sleep. I believe that her psyche had been disturbed. Penny was experiencing strong emotions about her life, although she said that she had no pictures or information of her life story.

The family history, not only for Penny but also her siblings and mother, was that it wasn't safe to talk about or recall the past. These unspoken taboos left Penny with no sense of self, so it was agreed that mum would join some of the sessions in order to help Penny put together a life story. Penny needed to increase her sense of self and self-esteem and needed to be able to balance her hysterical/happy feelings and her fear. Family photos were brought to the next four sessions, and by using the family tree, Penny and her mother shared memories of their past homes, Christmases and holidays. Penny's mother became upset at times during this process, and Penny was sad for her mother, highlighting their intense closeness. Individual counselling was offered to Penny's mother, which she accepted.

What is really interesting about this case is that Penny was able to explore her issues through the metaphor of flowers. My hope is that when Penny meets the crises that the other family members create, she will be able to have the choice to stand on the outside and not accept the role of supporting in order to be nurtured. Like the sunflower in the very first session, she must speak up for herself within her family.

Penny's case clearly shows that it is not always possible for play therapy to have a great effect in changing the outer world experiences of a child. Yet it is possible to explore choices for a different way to behave or approach problems, and to provide a greater opportunity for finding solutions.

Gill (1991) suggests that it is important to provide the 'opportunity to help process the painful and the frightening events before the defence mechanisms solidify in the personality, causing denial, avoidance, behavioural or play re-enactments, or a variety of symptomatic behaviours' (p.194).

Conclusion

Play therapy is an exploration between a therapist and a child of the child's life events. It can be child-centred or focused, or a mixture of both, with the child giving direction through the medium of play. The child needs to understand boundaries within the play therapy room and the role of the therapist. It is important to explore the areas a child is happy to share with others outside the room and any issues the therapist feels are important for carers to know. Play therapy is an area for unconditional regard, respect and honesty. Play therapy is a moment of time for children living in a complex environment. Through the play, I can help children to discover ways of having a voice. It is important for the child's significant others to understand that the process of play therapy is therapeutic and not investigative, as I believe this could cause further abuse (Cattanach, 1992).

Daniel developed a creative response to high levels of anxiety. He made a two-sided picture which could alert his mother to his feelings when he was unable to verbalise them. Daniel's mother learned to respond accordingly. Rebecca has learned to deal with fear through humour. Her stepfather has left, and her mother became stronger and more protective. Tony began to deal with the dark side of his family, and placed the responsibility with them rather than holding it all himself. Unfortunately, his mother could not handle this development and terminated the play therapy, verbalising this by rejecting the need for further play. Peter's mother left home, and the change in his circumstances meant that his play showed other relationships developing, and the change in his responses within those relationships.

Children reveal themselves gradually, at a pace they can tolerate. The therapist must be patient, attend to small nuances and allow children to communicate through the props, stories or pictures which stimulated them.

The purpose of the play therapy process for the child is to provide a corrective and repairing experience. This process allows the child to consciously understand traumatic events and tolerate them, within the rewarding relationship. The child needs to feel safe and accepted, which will encourage trust and a sense of well-being that can be held in the mind, and which will sustain the child in the future.

References

Association of Play Therapists (1995) *Association of Play Therapists Newsletter*, 3, p.1.

Cattanach, A. (1992) *Play Therapy with Abused Children*, London: Jessica Kingsley.

Freud, S. (1955) 'Beyond the pleasure principle', in Strachey, J. (ed.) *The Standard Edition of the Complete Psychological Works of Sigmund Freud*, Vol.XVIII: 1920–1922, London: Hogarth Press, pp.7–64.

Gill, E. (1991) *The Healing Power of Play*, New York: Guilford Press.

Grainger, R. (1990) *Drama and Healing*, London: Jessica Kingsley.

Lowenfeld, M. (1950) 'The nature and use of the Lowenfeld world technique in work with children and adults', *Journal of Psychology*, 30, pp.325–31.

Oaklander, V. (1978) *Windows to Our Children*, Highland, NY: The Gestalt Journal Press.

Terr, L. (1983) *Play Therapy*, New York: Wiley Interscience.

Terr, L. (1990) *Too Scared to Cry*, New York: Basic Books.

10 What can group therapy offer?

Jason Maratos

Introduction: Self-psychology and attachment theory

Our understanding of anxiety has been greatly enhanced by the contributions of two major and new schools of thought: those of self-psychology (Kohut, 1971; for a brief review, see Maratos, 1988) and of attachment theory (Bowlby, 1969, 1973, 1980). These two theories complement each other in many ways (Maratos, 1986), and in relation to the subject of anxiety more specifically.

Attachment theory helped us understand the origin of anxiety experienced by a person on moving away from another person (originally a mother or other agent who made their position a 'secure base'); Bowlby alerted us to the nature of separation anxiety. Self-psychology made us aware of the origin of anxiety arising from the proximity of one person to another.

Anxiety of separation and anxiety of proximity

Readers of this chapter will be immediately aware that it is impossible for one to separate the anxiety of separation from the anxiety of proximity; the two concepts are separate only conceptually, and for reasons of study; in reality, moving away and getting close are different aspects of the same experience. Moving away from mother would not generate the feelings that it does if the same move was not bringing the child closer to an 'other' person, animal or even place. Furthermore, we need not forget that moving away from a secure base and getting near to other people (and even places) is often, in a psychologically healthy person, a source of pleasurable excitement.

Separation and proximity generate pleasurable excitement as well

Throughout life, healthy individuals go through phases, one close to the other, of enjoying the security of a trusted base, and soon after, of seeking the excitement of new encounters with new places and with new people. Healthy toddlers will (for a brief period) leave their mothers and seek the company of other toddlers, and even that of other adults. Healthy adolescents will not only seek to be away from their parents, but will consider as nothing short of disaster to have their 'secure base' with them when they are with their girlfriend or boyfriend. A phobic girl patient of mine surprised herself when, soon after beginning psychotherapy, she discovered that she wanted to be away from her home and her parents, and even became irritated with their questions as to whether she would 'really' be alright without them.

Fluidity of life needs to be matched with change in self and attachments

The fortunate person who feels that they have a secure base (the securely-attached individual) can maintain the relationship with this 'base', distance themselves from it for a while, and return later as and when it is appropriate. Leaving does not mean abandoning; what I refer to here is the need for fluidity and change in relationships, so that they match the fluidity and perpetual change of the individual's growth and development. The healthy adolescent is not content to have a relationship with their parents which has the quality and characteristics of the relationship of a toddler. It is not only the adolescent who will seek this change; their parents will also allow and encourage it. Relationships need to keep pace with the changes in individuals.

In parent–child systems, fluidity needs to be fostered by parents

We are all too well aware of those parent–child systems in which relationships fail to adapt to the development of either parents or children, the families in which parents hold children back and in which children are too fearful to experiment. In such families, toddlers behave and/or are treated as babies, adolescents are treated as toddlers, and young adults behave as late adolescents.

Discrimination versus blind trust or paranoia

But what is the healthy way of moving on? Does 'healthy' mean the development of blind trust in the 'world' or 'the other'? Not at all; blind *anything* is dysfunctional and dangerous – blind trust as well as blind suspicion. The all-trusting person is simply naive, while the all-mistrusting is paranoid. The healthy individual is able to approach each situation, judging it accurately; if it is a dangerous situation, it is handled as such, and differently from a safe one. The healthy and mature individual is able to *discriminate* – is able to differentiate one situation from the other, and one person from another. (It is a shame that this extremely useful word has been abused and is now taken to mean 'to discriminate against', with the absurd consequence of whole government departments adopting 'anti-discriminatory' policies, thus expecting their employees to be unable to detect any difference between staff or clients!)

Safety and dangerousness are subjective notions

But trust and dangerousness are not independent concepts; they cannot stand on their own; situations are not equally dangerous or safe for all. Crossing the road may be safe for one 3-year-old, but not for another; crossing one road may be safe, but not crossing another. Trust and dangerousness depend on the ability of the person to deal with the situation.

Another factor that complicates matters even further is the fact that trust is based on perception of the ability of the self to cope with the situation, as well as on the perception of the difficulty and the intent (friendly or otherwise) of the other, and neither perception of the ability of the self nor the perception of the intent of the other are infallible. In fact, both are based on the individual's earlier experiences. A girl who finds that she is welcomed by other pupils at school will have a different perception of her self from another who is shunned by her peers. (The word 'earlier' is used here instead of the word 'early' to reaffirm Bowlby's contention that it is not only the first experiences which are important, but later ones as well.)

Bowlby: Development continues throughout life

One of Bowlby's major contributions is the notion that development continues throughout life, and that it is not fixed (in emotional terms) in the first days or years of life. It is difficult to comprehend how some therapists work, offering a contemporary experience to their clients, while at the same time claiming that contemporary or later experiences do not play a major role in a person's person. lity development. It is the intensity and the relevance of an experience that makes it therapeutic, not the profession of the persons involved in it. Group therapy is based on this premise, and we will return to this point later on.

Reasonable sense of security and of self

So what does a child need in order to approach life without undue anxiety and without being foolhardy? What does a child need in order to be able to explore the world, to be able to apply themself to work and to develop psychologically?

What seems to be an essential minimum is a reasonable sense of security and a reasonable sense of self. ('Reasonable' is used here in the same sense that Winnicott used the term 'good enough': something that is not perfect but realistically attainable.)

The imperfect is the ideal

It may sound paradoxical, but in this case, the reasonable (and imperfect) is the ideal, while the ideal would be dangerous and wrong, and therefore quite unreasonable. 'Reasonable' means not only humanely acceptable (rather than rigidly seeking a harsh perfection); it implies that imperfections are part of nature, and should not be seen as unbearable faults. Reason does not imply complacency; on the contrary, the person with a reasonable sense of self and reasonable sense of attachment is more free to improve and grow than someone who is burdened with feelings of inadequacy (in comparison with an idealised image of the self) and insecurity (in comparison with a hoped-for perfect security of attachment). Some awareness of the failings of the self and some appreciation of the uncertainty of the world are not only essential for survival, but also healthy stimulants for psychological growth.

The inevitability of change – of attachments

The person (young or old) who lives with the intention to adhere to and to preserve earlier forms of attachment and earlier forms of self is fighting a losing battle; the objective of maintaining early forms of attachment and of self is simply unattainable (as well as undesirable). This person will experience life as a series of attacks on what they aim to preserve. It is because they aim to preserve an earlier self and attachments that they will experience the normal encounters of life as attacks rather than opportunities for growth and enjoyment.

The anxious toddler who wishes to preserve the infantile mother–child relationship will approach playgroup with fear; the presence of other children will be perceived as a threat to the child's infantile relationship. The fact remains that peer relationships are indeed a threat to infantile mother–child relationships; it is their presence that will contribute to the healthy toddler's progress from psychological infancy to toddlerhood, and therefore the eventual 'death' of the infantile attachment. In the healthy individual, the infantile attachment is gradually and happily replaced by the age-appropriate toddler–mother and toddler–peer relationships. The healthy child and the healthy parent will be looking forward towards growth, while the dysfunctional family will be looking backwards towards preserving the past. For them, the inevitable change will be a source of sadness for the loss of the past and a source of anxiety and anger, because it is bringing undesirable changes.

The inevitability of change – of selves

What is valid for attachments is also true for the 'self'. In clinical practice, we come across individuals of any age who wish to preserve their earlier selves. In therapy, this wish manifests itself as resistance; in relationships, it comes across as rigidity and intransigence. People who wish to preserve their earlier self will not change in response to feedback from relationships; they will maintain that they are right and that the others are wrong. This defensive stance will be perceived as arrogance, and will often offend. The offence often leads to traumatic relationships, with hostility which can lead to the elaboration of paranoid systems of ideas.

The pathology I am describing here has been referred to as 'pathological narcissism'. Healthy individuals will be open to adopt, as their own, qualities and characteristics of others which are functional and age-appropriate, and will abandon, without much pain, features which are no longer appropriate or are dysfunctional. In this way, they will become richer as persons, and because of their wealth of qualities, also more distinct as individuals. By adopting qualities of others, they become better selves, and selves different from their own earlier ones. Followers of the object-relations theory will recognise here the concepts of introjection and identification, while self-psychologists will recognise the notion of self-objects.

Narcissists will build a fortress around their primitive early self, draw the bridge, drop the portcullis and fight against any alien intrusions. They will live in fear of these aliens, but in defending themselves against them, they will also starve themselves and stunt their growth. The further away their psychological growth gets from their chronological, the more pathological they will be, and the more terrified. Their poor, rigid, brittle and out-of-context selves will be in real danger of breakdown and, by now, their fear will have a realistic basis, because persons with such personality structure run a high risk of breakdown – psychological as well as physical.

Those who have followed the argument of this chapter will be aware that, in brief, anxiety can be seen as a component of an attachment disorder and a disturbance of the self.

Group therapy

Group therapy has many forms and means different things to different people. I will refer here to group therapy as described by S.H. Foulkes (1948, 1964; Foulkes & Anthony, 1957) and developed by his disciples, who formed the Institute of Group Analysis and the Group Analytic Society in London. Those interested in this school of thought who wish to follow the developments in this field will be rewarded if they look up the society's journal, *Group Analysis*. It is beyond the scope of this chapter to mention more than some of the basic principles.

Group therapy is an experience; by this, we mean that it is more than a cognitive exercise. The group experience is a part of the participant's real life. It is a powerful experience, to be compared and contrasted to the other (earlier and more recent) life experiences.

An experience is made up of an event and of the meaning that is attributed to it:

Experience = Event + Meaning

The event is the actual interaction between peers in the group. The interaction is real and meaningful. What one person says to the other is important within the context of the group. In this context, communications are acts, and acts of commission or omission are communications. The physical presence or absence of the person in the group session, the talk or the silence, the smile or the tear, the laugh or the shout, are all communications and acts which are laden with meaning.

The presence of the group conductor fulfils two main functions: the first is that it maintains the interaction within safe boundaries (a threatening group is an inhibiting group or a dying group), and the second is that it ensures that the meaning that is given to the experience is accurate. The natural tendency of all of us is to interpret the new on the basis of old experience. Naturally, those who are 'bitten' will anticipate being 'bitten' when they encounter new 'dogs'. The fact remains that many dogs do not bite. The traumatised child will interpret the new life events through the only 'eyes' they have – the traumatised 'eyes', through their own experience. The various schools of therapy have given different titles to this function of logical mental activity, and the prevailing term is that used by psycho-analysis: transference. This misinterpretation of the experience takes place not only towards the group conductor (who is seen initially as an image of a traumatising parent), but also (and this feature is unique to group therapy) towards the other group members.

The participant of the therapeutic group is able to understand that the current interactions do not have the same meaning as the 'other' intra-familial or earlier ones. Psycho-analysts refer to this phenomenon as 'transference resolution'. The earlier experiences are not invalidated; it is the new ones that are no longer distorted. The patient/client is developing an ability to discriminate events (new from old) and people (well-intentioned from mal-intentioned).

This ability to discriminate makes it possible for the patient/client to move away from paranoia (in which the world is seen as a hostile place) and from a naive belief in an idealised benevolence of humankind. Being able to discriminate does not imply a tendency to discriminate *against*; on the contrary, those who discriminate against are often unable to discriminate between the various members of a group, and treat all of them as if they were one. Indiscriminate treatment of a group who share a common feature (same sex, culture, race or religion, to mention a few) is either naive idealisation or an abusive 'ism' (racism, sexism, etc.).

The experience of the therapeutic group will not only enable the participants to have more accurate perceptions of the world, but it is a formative experience for their own selves.

Development of aspects of the self through group therapy

During the group sessions, just as a person's view of the world is being challenged, so is their view of themselves. The group members meet only within the sessions, they are not related to each other and are not dependent on each other in any way outside the group. The interactions within the group will not have any direct consequences in their ordinary life.

But, one may ask, how can we talk of 'interactions' and of 'events' within the group, when one of the principles of groupwork is that there is no action, no touch, no giving and taking, and no eating or smoking. Is it not 'just talk'? Is it different from a discussion group? There is a vast difference between an experiential group and a discussion group. An example may illustrate the difference better than a long explanation.

Talking about trust between young people arises from personal feelings but constitutes a discussion. Telling a member of the group that you trust them to keep a secret is an act, and the interaction between these two people (and the group within which such an act takes place) constitutes an event. Once this event is given meaning/significance, it forms the basis of a new experience: the experience of having been trusted; the experience that 'there are some people in the world who think something positive about me'; the experience that 'I am trustworthy.'

Events in the group need not be based only on verbal communications; a smile, a nod, attentiveness in silence, sharing a laugh, sinking in the chair or even falling asleep are significant acts, significant events, which have an impact on the whole membership of the group (though to a different extent for each member). Meaning to these events is not given primarily by the conductor through interpretations; meaning is arrived at through 'work' between the group members. The conductor and the group work at providing the context in which new meaning can be arrived at. It is this meaning that will transform these simple events into significant experiences.

Through such numerous and varied experiences, group participants will develop new, more accurate, more mature and more up-to-date views of themselves. Accurate perception does not equal high regard; 'accurate' means that the perception of strengths and weaknesses, qualities and skills will be seen from a more accurate/realistic perspective.

But, you may wonder, what is therapeutic about being aware of one's limitations or even negative qualities? This is where group therapy makes a unique contribution: the group provides the forum for (a) acceptance of limitations and (b) development of the self – again, within realistic boundaries. In the days before the development of self-psychology, Foulkes called this function of the group 'ego training in action'; if he were alive today, I am convinced he would be referring to 'self-training in action'.

An additional gain from group therapy (and again unique to this form of treatment) is that the participants have acquired all these benefits through interaction with peers. They have learned how to learn from interaction with others like themselves, even though the others had difficulties, problems or even undesirable characteristics. This is a skill that can stay with them, and can be a great asset to them throughout their lives. Upon leaving the group, they have not completed their therapy, they have begun a new life of emotional growth, which they can achieve through interaction with their natural environment.

The role of group therapy in the treatment of anxiety: Case example

Jackie was 13 years old when she was referred to my clinic. The referral from her general practitioner was of high quality and very informative:

> This bright young lady is presently at the High School [in a nearby town – the educational system locally selects children at the age of 12 for high/grammar school or upper-school education]. Since starting at the school she has had problems adjusting to the pace there and difficulty in making friends. Over recent months it has got to the stage where she is being almost ostracised by her friends because of her rather bizarre behaviour at times. She has, over the last month, started to develop paranoid feelings. She has had a host of physical complaints for which she has always attended the school matron. She has expressed to her that she feels that she is being watched all the time. She has had counselling at school, who are very concerned about her, but this has not helped the situation at all.
>
> She is a very quiet, introspective, usually shy girl and I think she has been very sheltered by her parents, who had her quite late in life after a big gap between their previous two children. Mother is finding the whole situation extremely stressful and difficult to cope with and there is obviously concern that she is beginning to develop psychotic symptoms and I would be most grateful for your opinion.

This referral contains the elements of an excellent psychiatric assessment of the child and of the family. It describes a child functioning on the borderline between neurosis and psychosis (the anxiety, the psycho-somatic complaints, the paranoid ideation). Such a clinical picture in an adult would justify the diagnosis of borderline character structure or borderline personality disorder; but in an adolescent, personality is (fortunately) much more fluid, and it is for this reason I refer here to the level at which she was functioning at that time. We were also given the information that individual counselling did not help at all. The family doctor also made the valid association with the family picture and the personality of the mother. Finally, he showed that he was aware of the seriousness of the prognosis.

A number of experienced therapists believe that group techniques are not suitable for seriously-disturbed children or adolescents, who, they feel, should be seen individually. The individual attention that Jackie had been given had not helped her, and we believed that only a new experience with peers could counteract her anxieties about peers, and about herself in relation to peers. We invited her to take part in a psychotherapy group which was already operating at my clinic, and we followed the verbal explanations with a letter setting some groundrules; we feel that a lot of what is said in the heat of an interview is often forgotten, and a letter is a useful reminder. The letter is addressed to the adolescent themself at the home address. It reads as follows:

Dear . . . . . .

I was pleased to meet you yesterday and to hear that you are still interested in joining our group for young people. I am taking the chance that this letter will reach you before Monday. As I told you, it confirms much of what we talked about when we met.

The group began in June of last year and following a break during August, resumed in September, meeting every Monday during term time from 4.15–5.30 p.m. The group is a forum where young people between the ages of 14 and 17 can meet regularly to explore attitudes, feelings and relationships. As professionals, we are naturally present but the main work of this group is carried out by its members. There is no formal agenda and the young members decide what they want to put their minds to.

The participants need to undertake to keep confidentiality and not discuss outside the group what has been said in the sessions. This will give all members freedom to discuss things that really matter to them without fear of gossip. It is unlikely that members of the group will know each other socially and we would encourage this to continue to be so, making it easier for members to observe the confidentiality and also share with the group things that they may not wish to discuss with their family, friends or neighbours.

We, as professionals, undertake to respect the confidentiality of the group regarding what happens and what is said in the group sessions although we would have to let your home know if you have not attended a session once you have become a member of the group.

You can continue as part of the group as long as you feel this helps you and you can leave when you feel ready to do so. It is best to discuss with the group your decision to leave and take into account what the group feels about your leaving. It is also useful to give yourself and the group some 'notice' about your leaving.

As you can see, joining a group of this kind can offer a great deal but it is also quite a commitment. It makes demands on you as it is a more adult way of sorting out difficulties and it depends a lot on your own contribution to it. There is, however, much to gain from this type of experience and Dr Maratos and I are pleased that you are joining the group and we look forward to seeing you on Monday.

Yours sincerely

Jason Maratos   Pippa Greenwood (Mrs)
Consultant Psychiatrist   Social Worker

Jackie's progress through the group can best be followed through some extracts from recordings of the group sessions.

Clive started the session by explaining his absence from the last group session due to examinations. Jim barged in like a bull in a china shop, and started interrogating Jackie. Jackie was near the brink, and in fact did cry, but also managed to compose herself and talk about the teasing that she was being subjected to on the way to and from school. Clive was becoming painfully aware that he was being left out, and the conductors intervened to bring some balance to the interaction. Clive was able to share with Jackie that he too was the subject of teasing, and shared with the group how he had managed to put a stop to it.

Jim's intrusive questioning became a warmer wish to understand Jackie's plight, and Jackie later on thanked him for his thoughtful interest in her. Jim was embarrassed and pleased with Jackie's compliment. Clive spoke of the difficulties that he was having at home, and Jim shared his own, and they experienced a feeling of empathy for each other.

Even by the end of one session, a warmth had developed between the three youngsters; they experienced a transition from a potentially fearful encounter to one of comradeship. They found themselves being valued by the others and this improved their feeling of value for themselves. Jackie, in particular, experienced that she was able to deal with the intrusive questioning of Jim, and that by responding with some confidence, she contributed to forming not a persecutory but a mutually-supportive relationship.

In the following week, the group began to explore more powerful feelings, their expression, and the negotiation with each other. They had clearly been moved (and freed) by Jackie's crying. Lois said that she would never cry in front of others, including the group. After some discussion, the group moved into an exploration of how they would handle their own and other people's violence. To some, this may seem like a change of topic. The conductors felt that the group was beginning to understand that feelings of violence (and violent acts) often follow and arise from feelings of hurt, and that it would be more useful for the group members to experience the association than for the conductors to interpret the apparent change of subject as defensive avoidance of feelings of hurt.

In the following session, Jim shared with the group his feelings of grief about the imminent death of an uncle of his. The other members tuned into his and their own feelings of grief and mourning, and in this way, numerous changes were achieved; they derived comfort from each other, they advanced their own resolution of mourning, they experienced being open and 'vulnerable' in front of their peers, and also experienced that allowing themselves to be 'vulnerable' can be an experience that not only does not undermine, but on the contrary, strengthens and brings people together.

In the sessions that followed, the group members explored their anxieties about their relationships with the opposite sex, and in particular how their experiences of interactions were partly of attraction and partly of confrontation and challenge. Jackie shared with the group new experiences of being bullied. The arrival of new members brought to the fore anxieties about trust and vulnerability within the group, both in the new members and the old. One new member had intense agoraphobic and claustrophobic symptoms; the members experienced some degree of anxiety similar to agoraphobia and claustrophobia, each to varying degree, and were able to overcome it (again, each one to different degree) in the context of the group. It was not so much the 'talking about it' and the thinking that goes with talking which contributed to the diminution of anxiety, but the actual experience of overcoming the anxiety experienced within the group that was therapeutic.

Continuity between sessions is evident sometimes, while other sessions appear to have their own, separate beginnings. This discontinuity sometimes gives the impression that the group operates at a psychotic level, and this may indeed be the case, as, for example, in the next session, which started as follows.

Jim began the session by saying that this would be his last group meeting. There was no comment from the other group members. Lois asked one of the conductors (J.M.) if it would be appropriate to share with other members of the group how their participation in the group made them feel. When she was encouraged to do so, she proceeded to tell Jackie that when Jackie frequently cried, Lois felt that she was 'attention-seeking'. Lois also felt that Jackie cried in order to stop others asking questions of her. The implication was that Jackie's crying was a manipulative, controlling act. This statement brought tears to Jackie's eyes, but she was able to explain that when she was upset, her eyes 'just welled-up'. Jackie then moved into some form of counter-offensive, and told Lois that crying might be for her what smoking was for Lois. In the interaction that followed, Jackie became more aware of how her distress was perceived by her peers, of how it influenced their feelings against her, and thus aggravated her relationships with them. Through the interaction, Jackie began to develop the ability to defend herself and show to her peers that she (through crying) was not abnormal or any less worthy a person compared with anyone else who had other ways of dealing with or manifesting their distress (as, for example, smoking). Having made progress in this respect, she then proceeded to exercise better control of how, when and to whom she showed her feelings.

The group went through periods of discomfort as, for example, when there were long silences (once for 20 minutes), when there was disagreement between members, and between members and the conductors, when defensive overtalking served a function of avoiding the live experience and of comforting tensions when they were too difficult to handle. There were also unhelpful influences when, for example, one fragile member 'dropped out' of the group, leaving the remaining members with mixed and troublesome feelings.

Conclusion

I hope to have given a brief account of the theoretical underpinning of one form of practice of group therapy for the treatment of anxiety in children and adolescents, and to have given a brief example illustrating how the theory 'works' in practice.

My own feeling about group therapy with children and adolescents is that it represents a territory which is very little explored, which is fascinating and powerful, and in which I will never be an expert, as there will always be so much more to learn. These very features make this kind of groupwork such an exciting field.

References

Bowlby, J. (1969) *Attachment and Loss, Vol.1: Attachment*, New York: Basic Books.
Bowlby, J. (1973) *Attachment and Loss, Vol.2: Separation, Anxiety and Anger*, New York: Basic Books.
Bowlby, J. (1980) *Attachment and Loss, Vol.3: Loss, Sadness and Depression*, New York: Basic Books.
Foulkes, S.H. (1948) *An Introduction to Group Analytic Psychotherapy*, London: Heinemann.
Foulkes, S.H. (1964) *Therapeutic Group Analysis*, London: Allen and Unwin.
Foulkes, S.H. & Anthony, E.J. (1957) *Group Psychotherapy: The Psychoanalytical Approach*, Harmondsworth: Penguin.
Kohut, H. (1971) *The Analysis of the Self*, New York: International Universities Press.
Maratos, J. (1986) 'Bowlby and Kohut: Where science and humanism meet', *Group Analysis*, 19, pp.303–9.
Maratos, J. (1988) 'Self psychology', *Current Opinion in Psychiatry*, 1, pp.284–8.

11 Pharmacotherapy of anxiety disorders

Anthony James

Introduction

The science of paediatric psychopharmacology is still in its infancy (see Gadow, 1992; Campbell & Cueva, 1995a, 1995b). This is particularly true of the pharmacological treatment of anxiety disorders, where research data are limited. Research to date has been beset by methodological problems, including: a confusing nosology; the high degree of comorbidity of anxiety disorders; a lack of validated clinical measures, and an interestingly high placebo response rate, which may mask drug effects (Puig-Antich et al., 1987). Partly as a result of this, there are no clear clinical guidelines for treatment. Nevertheless, there are some interesting developments, especially in the pharmacological treatment of obsessive-compulsive disorder.

Anxiety states

Anxiety disorders are relatively common. Kashani and Orvaschel (1988) report that in a community sample of adolescents aged 14–16 years, 17.3% met criteria for one or two DSM-III anxiety disorders. With the added criterion of 'significant impairment requiring treatment', the reported rate dropped to 8.7%. This is very similar to the rate of 8.9% reported for children aged 7–11 in a paediatric setting (Costello, 1989), which included: 4.1% with separation disorder, 4.6% with overanxious disorder, 1% with social phobia, 1.6% with avoidant disorder and 1.2% with agoraphobia. Obsessive-compulsive disorder was initially thought to be a rare illness; however, recent reports suggest weighted prevalence rates of 1% for current episodes and 1.9% for lifetime disorder (Flament et al., 1988) – evidence consistent with a relapsing and chronic course.

167

There is a large comorbidity with anxiety disorders. Bernstein (1991) found that 61% of children diagnosed as having anxiety disorder also met criteria from major depressive disorder (MDD), and that children with high levels of anxiety recorded more depressive symptoms. Similarly, 81% of children with major depressive disorder received a diagnosis of separation anxiety disorder.

In a naturalistic study of 275 children of parents with affective disorders, anxiety was shown to be a protracted illness with relapses. An estimate of the lifetime duration of illness suggested 46% would be ill for at least eight years (Keller et al., 1992).

Any proposed treatment is therefore set against the background of relatively common disorders, some of which – separation anxiety disorder and school refusal – occur only in children and adolescents, although these may bear some similarity to anxiety disorders and agoraphobia in adulthood. The natural history points, in a proportion of cases, to prolonged impairment.

Treatment principles

To encourage the appropriate use of pharmacological treatments for anxiety disorders, treatment should be based, as far as possible, upon well-documented principles, and guided by research findings.

1   *Diagnosis*: This should conform to DSM-IV or ICD-10 criteria. Anxiety disorders share a large comorbidity with depressive disorders, which makes accurate diagnosis essential.

2   *Formulation*: This should involve an accurate appraisal of all the psychosocial factors – school, family, etc. – including the psychodynamics of the therapy and counter-transference issues (Schowalter, 1989).

3   *Adequate trial of psychological treatments*: There is increasing evidence that behavioural and cognitive-behavioural treatments are effective in: panic disorder (Kane & Kendell, 1989), school refusal (Blagg & Yule, 1984) and obsessive-compulsive disorder (March et al., 1994; March, 1995). These should be attempted first for several reasons: although psychological treatments may initially be slightly more expensive in terms of therapists' time, if the patient is able to learn the method and administer it themselves or with the aid of a co-therapist, the longer-term

treatment course may be reduced, and the patient may be left with an increased sense of mastery, rather than dependence upon medication. The side effects of medication are clearly avoided.

4 *Appropriate use of medication*: A trial of drug treatment should involve medication, given at sufficient dosage and for a sufficient length of time, bearing in mind the knowledge of drug side effects and the effect of the medication upon the developing brain. Unfortunately, data upon the latter are scarce.

Neurochemistry

This subject is well reviewed by Rogeness et al. (1992). There are over 30 neurotransmitters, of which the three foremost are dopamine (DA), noradrenaline (NA), and 5 hydroxy-tryptamine (5 HT). Gray (1982) has proposed a neurobiochemical model of anxiety which involves the septo-hippocampal system. The 'Papez' circuit begins in the limbic cortex (cingulate gyrus) and projects to the entorhinal cortex (temporal lobe). From the hippocampus, the circuit goes via the mamilliary bodies to the thalamus and back to the limbic cortex. Neuronal activity is modulated by the NA neurones from the locus coeruleus and 5 HT neurones from the raphe nuclei. The hippocampus is seen as the area of integration.

All three neurotransmitters are involved in 'tuning' the neuronal systems. There is a dynamic balance between the behavioural facilitatory system (BFS), mainly a dopaminergic system, and the behavioural inhibitory system (BIS), which depends upon noradrenergic activity, with additional regulation from the serotonergic (5 HT) projections from the median raphe (Gray, 1982, 1987).

Developmental factors

Evidence from cerebro-spinal fluid (CSF) studies suggest developmental changes in dopamine and serotonergic (5 HT) systems, with levels of the metabolites homo-vanillic acid (HVA) and 5 hydroxy indole acetic acid (5 HIAA) decreasing with age (see Rogeness et al., 1992). In contrast, the levels of noradrenaline metabolites (3 methoxy-4 hydroxy-phenylglycol – MHPG) remain stable after eight to nine months. The evidence suggests increasing central nervous system inhibition with age. Preliminary evidence from CSF studies of mother-deprived and mother-reared infant monkeys suggests that early psychosocial factors can affect the development of the NA system. These changes can be permanent and affect adult behaviour (Kraemer et al., 1989).

Separation anxiety, school phobia and overanxious disorder

Double-blind placebo-control studies of the drug treatment of school refusal and separation anxiety have yielded increasingly equivocal results. Gittelman-Klein and Klein (1971; 1973) treated 6–14-year-olds with behavioural counselling and imipramine (100–200 mg per day) for six weeks. Imipramine was superior to placebo after six weeks. Although children returning to school did not necessarily feel better, they were less fearful, had less physical complaints and were less depressed. Berney et al. (1981) treated school refusers aged 9–15, out of school for an average of six months, with clomipramine (40–75 mg per day). They found placebo and clomipramine equally effective in aiding school return. The two studies were not strictly comparable, as the latter patients were out of school longer and experienced different psychosocial interventions. Crucially, the dose of antidepressant was lower, an important factor given the evidence that children and adolescents metabolise tricyclic antidepressants (TCAs) more rapidly than adults (Wilens et al., 1992).

Bernstein et al. (1990) failed to demonstrate the effectiveness over placebo of either imipramine (150–200 mg per day) or alprazolam (0.75–4 mg per day) in treating severely symptomatic school refusers. Both alprazolam and imipramine did, however, reduce depressive symptoms. Similarly, Klein et al. (1992) could not replicate their initial positive findings: approximately 50% of patients with separation anxiety improved on either imipramine or placebo.

Fluoxetine, a serotonergic re-uptake inhibitor (SSRI), was reported as moderately-to-markedly effective in reducing anxiety symptoms in an open study of 21 children and teenagers with social phobias, separation anxiety and overanxious disorder (Birmaher et al., 1994). However, other classes of drugs, such as benzodiazepines, have not been shown to be particularly effective. Although earlier open trials of chlordiazepoxide indicated considerable improvement (Kraft et al., 1965), later controlled trials failed to show any benefit over placebo of alprazolam or clonazepam, and there were considerable side effects, including drowsiness and a risk of drug abuse or addiction (Simeon et al., 1992; Graae et al., 1994). A single case study (Kranzler, 1988) and one open trial (Kutchner et al., 1992) have been reported on the efficacy of Buspirone, a 5 HT-1 agonist, in the treatment of overanxious disorder.

The low incidence of symptomatic panic disorder in children and adolescents is cited as a reason for the lack of controlled trials in this population (Ambrosini et al., 1993). The case studies available indicate possible benefit from the use of benzodiazepines (Biederman, 1987) and tricyclic antidepressants (Ballenger et al., 1989).

Obsessive-compulsive disorder (OCD)

Two double-blind placebo-controlled trials of clomipramine in children and adolescents have demonstrated significant improvement in obsessive-compulsive symptoms (Flament et al., 1985; DeVeaugh-Geiss et al., 1992). Flament et al. (1985) noted a 46% average improvement in obsessive-compulsive symptoms in adolescents aged 10–18 treated with doses of up to 3 mg/kg clomipramine for five weeks. Interestingly, improvement was noted not only in symptom severity, but also in the lessening of symptom interference in daily life. Riddle et al. (1992) report a small trial of 14 children aged 8–15 with OCD, treated with fluoxetine (20 mg per day) for 20 weeks. A reduction of obsessive-compulsive symptomatology of 30–45% was obtained. The drug, on the whole, was well tolerated, although some complained of agitation and insomnia; one described suicidal ideation with an increase in self-harming behaviour, necessitating stoppage. Evidence is also accruing that other SSRIs, such as fluvoxamine, are beneficial in OCD (Apter et al., 1994); further double-blind studies are awaited.

In obsessive-compulsive disorder, there seems to be good evidence for the efficacy of serotonergic antidepressants, which contrasts with a lack of efficacy for noradrenergic antidepressants (Leonard et al., 1989). In line with this, Hanna et al. (1991) demonstrated that adolescents with OCD treated with clomipramine showed an initial increase in prolactin levels, which decreased in the last four weeks of treatment. The decline in prolactin levels was positively correlated with a favourable outcome, and negatively correlated with the duration of illness. This was interpreted as an adaptive decrease in the responsiveness of serotonergic receptors following clomipramine treatment.

A question raised by these findings, given the chronic and relapsing nature of moderate-to-severe OCD, is: what is the length of treatment? Unfortunately, reliable data for this age group are not yet available. If a parallel is drawn with the sometimes related disorder of depression, one could argue for an initial treatment course of six to nine months, with re-introduction of medication at times of stress or particular vulnerability. The long-term effects of these medications remain to be determined, but one must be concerned, particularly with an immature brain. This would, perhaps, argue for a treatment model that uses a combination of medication, at least initially, and targeted psychological interventions.

Side effects

The tricyclic antidepressants have important side effects, besides the anticholinergic effects of dry mouth, dizzinesss, blurred vision, etc. The most common cardio-vascular effects are tachycardia and postural hypotension. Related electrocardiogram (ECG) changes include: lengthened PR interval, QRS-widening and QT-lengthening (Ryan et al., 1987; Wilens et al., 1993). Ryan et al. (1987) found that once-daily dosage had minimal effects on the ECG parameters compared to three-times-per-day dosage regimes. The ECG changes were only modestly related to TCA levels (Wilens et al., 1993). Current opinion suggests routine monitoring of TCA levels, and a baseline ECG and further ECGs after dosage adjustment, especially if the daily dose is 3 mg/kg or greater (Wilens et al., 1993). Tricyclic antidepressants should be prescribed with caution, as overdosage can be lethal from cardiac and neurological effects.

Serotonin re-uptake inhibitors may initially increase agitation and insomnia, and occasionally cause akathisia. A rare serotonergic syndrome, secondary to excessive serotonin release, has been described, with hyperreflexia, restlessness, hypertension, delirium and convulsions. More common side effects of nausea and headaches are reported, but often resolve with continued administration. Migraine may be precipitated in potential sufferers. The SSRIs have been implicated in increasing suicidal ideation and self-harming behaviour (King et al., 1991), but this is rare, occurring in the setting of increasing agitation, dysphoria and akathisia (Power & Cowen, 1992). An advantage of SSRIs is their relative safety in overdosage, an especially important factor in impulsive self-harming adolescents (for a review of side effects, see Ambrosini et al., 1993).

Benzodiazepines should be prescribed in time-limited courses to prevent the risk of dependence. Limited data are available on the side effects of Buspirone, but there is a report of psychotic changes in the mental state of two children treated with this drug (Soni & Weintraub, 1992).

Conclusions

As yet, no specific recommendations can be made for the psychopharmacological treatment of the anxiety disorders – separation anxiety, overanxious disorder, etc. – although TCAs and SSRIs may be beneficial in reducing symptoms, particularly depressive symptoms. In contrast, in the case of moderate-to-severe OCD, serotonergic antidepressants (SSRIs) offer a valuable treatment option, backed by research data.

References

Ambrosini, P.J., Bianchi, M.D., Rabinovich, H. & Elia, J. (1993) 'Antidepressant treatments in children and adolescents, II: Anxiety, physical, and behavioral disorders', *Journal of the American Academy of Child and Adolescent Psychiatry*, 32(3), pp.494–500.

Apter, A., Ratzoni, G., King, R.A., Weizman, A., Iancu, I., Binder, M. & Riddle, M. (1994) 'Fluvoxamine open-label treatment of adolescent inpatients with obsessive-compulsive disorder or depression', *Journal of the American Academy of Child and Adolescent Psychiatry*, 33(3), pp.342–8.

Ballenger, J.C., Carek, D.J., Steele, J.J. & Cornish-McTighe, D. (1989) 'Three cases of panic disorder with agoraphobia in children', *American Journal of Psychiatry*, 141, pp.363–9.

Berney, T., Kolvin, I., Bhate, S.R., Garside, R.F., Jeans, J., Kay, B. & Scarth, L. (1981) 'School phobia: A therapeutic trial with clomipramine and short-term outcome', *British Journal of Psychiatry*, 138, pp.110–18.

Bernstein, G.A. (1991) 'Comorbidity and severity of anxiety and depressive disorders in a clinic sample', *Journal of the American Academy of Child and Adolescent Psychiatry*, 30(1), pp.43–50.

Bernstein, G.A., Garfinkel, B.D. & Borchardt, C.M. (1990) 'Comparative studies of pharmacotherapy for school refusal', *Journal of the American Academy of Child and Adolescent Psychiatry*, 29(5), pp.773–81.

Biederman, J. (1987) 'Clonazepam in the treatment of pre-pubertal children with panic-like symptoms', *Journal of Clinical Psychiatry*, 48(Supplement), pp.38–41.

Birmaher, B., Waterman, G.S., Ryan, N., Cully, M., Balach, L., Ingram, J. & Brodsky, M. (1994) 'Fluoxetine for childhood anxiety disorders', *Journal of the American Academy of Child and Adolescent Psychiatry*, 33(7), pp.993–9.

Blagg, N.R. & Yule, W. (1984) 'The behavioural treatment of school refusal: A comparative study', *Behaviour Research and Therapy*, 22, pp.119–27.

Campbell, M. and Cueva, J.E. (1995a) 'Psychopharmacology in child and adolescent psychiatry: A review of the past seven years – I', *Journal of the American Academy of Child and Adolescent Psychiatry*, 34, pp.1,124–32.

Campbell, M. and Cueva, J.E. (1995b) 'Psychopharmacology in child and adolescent psychiatry: A review of the past seven years – II', *Journal of the American Academy of Child and Adolescent Psychiatry*, 34, pp.1,262–72.

Costello, E.J. (1989) 'Child psychiatric disorders and their correlates: A primary care pediatric sample', *Journal of the American Academy of Child and Adolescent Psychiatry*, 28(6), pp.851–8.

DeVeaugh-Geiss, J., Moroz, G., Biederman, J., Cantwell, D., Fontaine, R., Greist, J.H., Reichler, R., Katz, R. & Landau, P. (1992) 'Clomipramine hydrochloride in childhood and adolescent obsessive-compulsive disorder: A multicentre trial', *Journal of the American Academy of Child and Adolescent Psychiatry*, 31(1), pp.45–9.

Flament, M.F., Rapoport, J.L., Berg, C.J. & Kilts, C. (1985) 'A controlled trial of clomipramine in childhood obsessive-compulsive disorder', *Psychopharmacology Bulletin*, 21, pp.150–2.

Flament, M.F., Whitaker, A., Rapoport, J.L., Davies, M., Berg, C.Z., Kalikow, K., Screery, W. & Schaffer, D. (1988) 'Obsessive-compulsive disorder in adolescence: An epidemiological study', *Journal of the American Academy of Child and Adolescent Psychiatry,* 27(6), pp.764–72.

Gadow, K.D. (1992) 'Pediatric psychopharmacotherapy: A review of recent research', *Journal of Child Psychology and Psychiatry,* 33, pp.153–96.

Gittelman-Klein, R. & Klein, D.F. (1971) 'Controlled imipramine treatment of school phobia', *Archives of General Psychiatry,* 25, pp.204–7.

Gittelman-Klein, R. and Klein, D.F. (1973) 'School phobia: Diagnostic considerations in the light of imipramine effects', *Journal of Nervous and Mental Disease,* 156, pp.196–215.

Graae, F., Milner, J., Rizotto, L. & Klein, R.G. (1994) 'Clonazepam in childhood anxiety disorders', *Journal of the American Academy of Child and Adolescent Psychiatry,* 33(3), pp.372–6.

Gray, J.A. (1982) *The Neuropsychology of Anxiety: An Enquiry into the Functions of the Septo-hippocampal System,* Oxford: Oxford University Press.

Gray, J.A. (1987) *The Psychology of Fear and Stress* (2nd edn), Cambridge: Cambridge University Press.

Hanna, G.L., McCracken, J.T. & Cantwell, D.P. (1991) 'Prolactin in childhood obsessive-compulsive disorder: Clinical correlates and response to clomipramine', *Journal of the American Academy of Child and Adolescent Psychiatry,* 30(2), pp.173–8.

Kane, M.T. & Kendall, P.C. (1989) 'Anxiety disorders in children: A multiple-base line evaluation of cognitive-behavioral treatment', *Behaviour Therapy,* 20, pp.499–508.

Kashani, J.H. & Orvaschel, H. (1988) 'Anxiety disorders in mid-adolescence: A community sample', *American Journal of Psychiatry,* 145(8), pp.960–4.

Keller, M.B., Lavori, P.W., Wunder, J., Beardslee, W.R., Schwartz, C.E. & Roth, J. (1992) 'Chronic course of anxiety disorders in children and adolescents', *Journal of the American Academy of Child and Adolescent Psychiatry,* 31(4), pp.595–9.

King, R.A., Riddle, M.A., Chappel, P.B., Hardin, M.T., Anderson, G.M., Lombroso, P. & Scahill, L. (1991) 'Case study: Emergence of self destructive phenomena in children and adolescents treated with fluoxetine treatment', *Journal of the American Academy of Child and Adolescent Psychiatry,* 30(2), pp.179–86.

Klein, R.G., Koplewicz, H.S. & Kanner, A. (1992) 'Imipramine treatment of children with separation anxiety disorder', *Journal of the American Academy of Child and Adolescent Psychiatry,* 31(1), pp.21–8.

Kraemer, G.W., Schmidt, D.E. & McKinney, W.T. (1989) 'A longitudinal study of the effect of different social rearing conditions on cerebro-spinal fluid norepinepherine and biogenic amine metabolites in rhesus monkeys', *Neuropsychopharmacology,* 2, pp.175–89.

Kraft, I.A., Ardali, C., Duffy, J.H., Hart, J.T. & Pearce, P. (1965) 'A clinical study of chlordiazepoxide in psychiatric disorders of children', *International Journal of Neuropsychiatry,* 1, pp.443–7.

Kranzler, H.R. (1988) 'Use of Buspirone in an adolescent with overanxious disorder', *Journal of the American Academy of Child and Adolescent Psychiatry,* 27(6), pp.789–90.

Kutchner, S.P., Reiter, S., Gardner, D.M. and Klein, R.G. (1992) 'The pharmacotherapy of anxiety disorders in children and adolescents', *Psychiatric Clinics of North America,* 15, pp.41–67.

Leonard, H.S., Swedo, S. & Rapoport, J.L. (1989) 'Treatment of obsessive-compulsive disorder with clomipramine and desimipramine: A double-blind crossover comparison in children and adolescents', *Archives of General Psychiatry*, 46, pp.1,088–92.

March, J.S. (1995) 'Cognitive-behavioural psychotherapy for children and adolescents with OCD: A review and recommendations for treatment', *Journal of the American Academy of Child and Adolescent Psychiatry*, 34(1), pp.17–18.

March, J.S., Mulle, K. & Herbel, B. (1994) 'Behavioral psychotherapy for children and adolescents with obsessive compulsive disorder: An open trial of a new proctol-driven treatment', *Journal of the American Academy of Child and Adolescent Psychiatry*, 33(3), pp.372–6.

Power, A.C. & Cowen, P.J. (1992) 'Fluoxetine and suicidal behaviour: Some clinical and theoretical aspects of a controversy', *British Journal of Psychiatry*, 161, pp.735–41.

Puig-Antich, J., Perel, J.M. & Lupatkin, W. (1987) 'Imipramine in prepubertal major depressive disorder', *Archives of General Psychiatry*, 44, pp.81–9.

Riddle, M.A., Scahill, L., King, R.A., Hardin, M.T., Anderson, G.M., Ort, S.I., Smith, C., Leckman, J.F. & Cohen, D.J. (1992) 'Double-blind, crossover trial of fluoxetine and placebo in children and adolescents with obsessive-compulsive disorder', *Journal of the American Academy of Child and Adolescent Psychiatry*, 31(6), pp.1,062–9.

Rogeness, G.A., Javors, M.A. & Pliska, S.R. (1992) 'Neurochemistry and child and adolescent psychiatry', *Journal of the American Academy of Child and Adolescent Psychiatry*, 31, pp.765–87.

Ryan, N.D., Puig-Antich, J. & Cooper, T. (1987) 'Relative safety of single versus divided dose imipramine in adolescent major depression', *Journal of the American Academy of Child and Adolescent Psychiatry*, 26, pp.400–6.

Schowalter, J.E. (1989) 'Psychodynamics and medication', *Journal of the American Academy of Child and Adolescent Psychiatry*, 28, pp.681–4.

Simeon, J.G., Ferguson, H.B., Knott, V., Roberts, N., Gauthier, B., Dubois, C. & Wiggins, D. (1992) 'Clinical, cognitive, and neurophysiological effects of alprazolam in children and adolescents with overanxious and avoidant disorders', *Journal of the American Academy of Child and Adolescent Psychiatry*, 31, pp.29–33.

Soni, P. & Weintraub, A.L. (1992) 'Case study: Buspirone-associated mental state changes', *Journal of the American Academy of Child and Adolescent Psychiatry*, 31, pp.1,098–9.

Wilens, T.E., Biederman, J., Baldessarini, R.J., Puopolo, P.R. & Flood, J.G. (1992) 'Developmental changes in serum concentrations of desipramine and 2-hydroxydesipramine during treatment with desipramine', *Journal of the American Academy of Child and Adolescent Psychiatry*, 31, pp.691–8.

Wilens, T.E., Biederman, J., Baldessarini, R.J., Puopolo, P.R. & Flood, J.G. (1993) 'Electrocardiographic effects of desipramine and 2-hydroxydesipramine in children, adolescents, and adults treated with desipramine', *Journal of the American Academy of Child and Adolescent Psychiatry*, 32, pp.798–804.

12 Hypnotherapy in children

Raj Kathane

Hypnotic techniques have been used with children for a very long time. Use of hypnosis can bring about unexpected and rewarding results in treatment of both physical and psychological conditions. This chapter should give the clinician a useful introduction to this very exciting field of the use of hypnotherapy with children.

History of hypnosis

Study of the history of medicine indicates that since antiquity, for as long as records have been kept, humankind has used the power of trance for healing numerous physical maladies. Since ancient times, in all cultures, primitive as well as sophisticated, spread across all the different parts of the world, people had recognised that trance or suggestion could have a very powerful and therapeutic effect, and this was one of the oldest of the medical and therapeutic arts.

Trance or hypnotic state may often be produced with surprising ease, which often allows charlatans and entertainers to misuse this very important therapeutic tool. In ancient days, and even now in many cultures around the world, trance is produced by the use of some elaborate rituals, such as a long walk to a temple of a god or goddess who is supposed to have some special magical powers, ritualistic singing and dancing, chanting or humming special sounds in a very monotonous manner, which may then be followed by an invocation from a person in authority in a special room or place. This atmosphere of mysticism and ceremony facilitated and heightened the induction of trance.

In the second century AD, the great Greek physician, Galen of Pergamum, taught the view that some invisible fluid filled the universe and flowed through the bodies and minds of all the people, and was responsible for good physical and mental health, and that sickness would be caused if this flow was interfered with. Around 1530, Paracelsus suggested that heavenly bodies have effects on people and can cause diseases. Around 1650, a German priest by the name of Kircher held the view that not only did stars and other heavenly bodies influence people, but people could influence each other by dint of magnetic powers. The Austrian physician, Franz Anton Mesmer (1733–1815), who graduated from Vienna, wrote a dissertation entitled *The Influence of The Planets on The Human Body.* In essence, this paper propounded that the universal, invisible fluid of Galen, which was influenced by the heavenly bodies, could be controlled and guided through the bodies of patients by the use of magnetised iron plates. Thus he embarked upon the practice of 'animal magnetism' in quite dramatic circumstances in his darkened consultation chambers in Vienna. He treated numerous patients who had otherwise been given up as untreatable and incurable by the medical authorities, often with very dramatic success. The resulting conflict with the established medical hierarchy in Vienna forced Mesmer to move to Paris, where he set up one of the most famous clinics in Europe, treating every conceivable type of illness. The term 'animal magnetism' later gave way to the term 'Mesmerism'. His theory of magnetic fluid was heavily criticised by the Franklin Commission in 1794. However, the clinical usefulness of his techniques continued to be proved by the English physician, John Elliotson, Physician and Professor at University College Hospital, London, and later by James Braid. The latter is credited with having coined the term 'hypnosis', from the Greek word *hypnos*, meaning sleep, because subjects in trances produced by Mesmer's techniques often appeared to be asleep.

In psychological theories, two schools of thought developed in France in the late nineteenth century: the Salpetriere School and the Nancy School. In Salpetriere, John-Claude Charcot (1734–1815) proposed that hypnosis could only occur in pathological states in predisposed hysterical individuals, whereas in Nancy, Ambroise Auguste Liebeault and Hippolyte Marie Bernheim first proposed the psychological theory including the concept of suggestibility which is crucial to hypnosis. In that sense, Liebeault may well be considered the father of modern hypnotism. However, the term itself was coined by Braid around 1843.

Later in the nineteenth century, Pierre Janet continued to investigate hypnosis, recognising that splitting of consciousness occurs, which then led to the theory of dissociation. Sigmund Freud (1856–1939), a brilliant neurologist by training, used hypnosis in his clinical practice. However, he was disappointed by the results and abandoned it in favour of free association, on which developed his school of psycho-analysis. This led to the decline of hypnosis in the early years of the twentieth century. Later, the work of people like Milton Erickson and Ernest Hilgard caused a revival of interest in it. In Britain, professionals interested in the use of hypnosis for medical and dental conditions formed organisations which have gone through a number of different name changes – the British Society for Clinical Hypnosis was formed in 1978; worldwide, there is also an International Society of Hypnosis, as well as a European Society of Hypnosis. As expected, hypnosis has also been investigated quite thoroughly, making use of some of the latest investigative tools at the disposal of modern medicine.

The use of hypnosis with children also dates back to very ancient times. It is generally accepted that using hypnotic trance is easier in children than in adults. Most of the above-mentioned great names in hypnosis had successfully treated children using the hypnotic techniques. A detailed account of Anton Mesmer's treatment using hypnosis in the case of a young girl called Marie-Therese Paradis, who had suffered from blindness since childhood and was considered untreatable by the medical specialists, and an account of Mesmer's success using hypnosis, can be found in Waxman (1989). Later, Breuer and Freud (1955) published the fascinating case history of 'Fraulein Anna O' (real name Bertha Pappenheim), who, although 21 when they treated her, had been ill since adolescence. Wester and O'Grady (1991) mention that Baldwin is credited with the first publication in 1891 specifically relating to child hypnotherapy, and that the first book on hypnotherapy with children was published by Ambrose (1961).

Thus hypnosis and hypnotherapy have come a very long way since the days of Galen.

Nature of and theories about hypnosis

Despite the fact that hypnosis has been used in clinical practice since time immemorial, and has been very extensively studied using the latest scientific investigative techniques and tools, even now controversy exists about the exact nature of hypnosis, its definition and how it works. Therefore, rather than attempting to give a precise definition of hypnosis, it may be more useful to mention what constitutes hypnosis.

Hypnosis is characterised by an altered state of consciousness or awareness. There is often intense concentration, which is focused inwards, while at the same time retaining a blunted sense of parallel awareness, which means that a hypnotised subject in the deepest trance will retain and register sensory awareness of what happens around them (such as noises in the other room), but will not be affected by these to the same extent as they would be if they were not in a trance. This is sometimes also called a 'reduction in general reality orientation' (GRO) (Shor, 1969). Such altered states of awareness or concentration while retaining some peripheral awareness can occur in many day-to-day, ordinary activities, such as driving a car or watching a movie in a cinema hall. During the hypnotic trance, there is greater access to the unconscious processes, and the subject's mind is more receptive to those suggestions which would be acceptable to them during a state of ordinary wakefulness (ego-syntonic suggestions). Powers of critical, rational analysis or evaluation, which are attributed to the conscious waking mind, are suspended or bypassed. The depth of the hypnotic state also fluctuates quite naturally, so that a subject in a deep trance may suddenly become more aware of their surroundings. The following characteristics are often associated with hypnosis, but are not exclusive or unique to it:

- general physical, musculo-skeletal relaxation;
- relaxation of mind;
- body immobility;
- varying degrees of dissociation, amnesia, hypermnesia, hypoanalgesia, analgesia or glove anaesthesia;
- ideo-motor activity;
- ideo-sensory activity;
- post-hypnotic suggestion;
- time lag and time distortion, either involving contraction of time or expansion of time;
- automatic writing;
- literalness;
- memory recall;
- catalepsy;
- age regression;
- hyperaesthesia.

In essence, hypnosis is a state of mind which one person induces in another, and during which, by making use of the intense concentration focused inwards, suggestions may be given by the 'hypnotist' to the 'subject', who, if the suggestion is ego-syntonic, is more likely to receive, accept and integrate that suggestion into their unconscious mind.

It is equally important to dispel some of the misconceptions about hypnosis. Hypnosis is not a state of simple sleep, and there is no loss of consciousness. Hypnotised subjects do not lose willpower or give away control to the hypnotherapist. They do not give away hidden secrets, and after the session, most people usually remember what happened during the trance. The person inducing hypnosis does not control the subject, or the subject's mind, and is unable to project into the mind of the subject anything that the subject does not want. Thus, as mentioned above, only ego-syntonic ideas will be received, and others are rejected.

EEG studies indicate that hypnosis is very different from sleep, and that the brain experiences a form of resting arousal.

Some theories of hypnosis

Bernheim proposed in 1886 that hypnosis occurs because of suggestion, as mentioned above. Charcot believed that hypnosis could only occur in people with abnormal or pathological inclinations, or a nervous constitution. This view is no longer tenable, because evidence suggests that at least 90% of the population can be hypnotised, thus making the phenomenon normative. A close connection has been shown between hypnotisability and suggestibility.

Pavlov suggested that hypnosis is a conditioned response, and the more often the trance is induced in a person, the easier it becomes to induce it, and also the depth increases, as would be suggested by the classical conditioning theory.

The neurophysiological theory, which uses findings from EEGs, concludes that a hypnotic trance is distinct from sleep, that it is more a form of resting arousal, but that there are subtle differences between restful waking with eyes closed, deep hypnotic trance and sleep: the alpha rhythm is identical between a light hypnotic trance and a non-hypnotised person relaxing with eyes closed; as hypnosis deepens, there is no change in the frequency, but a reduction in the voltage occurs, and if specific suggestion of sleep is given, then the frequency will diminish, with a concurrent increase in voltage, thus producing a typical sleep EEG recording (see Waxman, 1989, for a more detailed description of other theories).

Children are more easily hypnotised than adults. Adult methods of inducing hypnotic trance can be used after age 14, but sometimes from the age of 12. Slightly different techniques are required between the ages of 7 and 12, but children as young as 4 or 5 can also be hypnotised. (These age ranges are somewhat flexible.)

The hypnotic process

General considerations

At the outset, it is important to point out that readers should not believe that it is possible to learn the induction of hypnotic trance, the various subtleties involved in this, and its use in the therapeutic process, whether in adults or in children, simply by reading a chapter like this. It is *imperative* to have a proper training, both in theory and practicum, from well-trained teachers, or by attending accredited courses organised by recognised professional bodies. The purpose of this article is to give an idea about hypnotherapy in general, and in relation to children specifically, and it assumes the reader's familiarity with the subject of hypnosis. For those who are not familiar with it, this article should serve to increase their curiosity and intellectual appetite regarding this subject. Interested readers are advised to refer to more authoritative texts on this subject, such as Erickson (1964), Haley (1986) and O'Hanlon and Hexum (1990), and others which are listed in the References.

It is most important to remember, whether working with adult subjects or children, that the hypnotherapist has no power over the subject, and no attempts should be made to abuse the trust that the subject, client or patient places in the hypnotherapist (practitioner) by ridiculing them, insulting, inappropriate touching or by any other means whatsoever. It is essential to maintain medical confidentiality.

As with all therapeutic processes, it is important to establish a good rapport with the client. In order to do this, the therapist should hold a thorough initial interview and obtain background information about the nature of the problem. Rapport can be enhanced by the therapist making complementary use of body language, using techniques called 'matching and leading', but these can only be learnt in properly-conducted teaching workshops. It is essential to establish the client's motivation in ridding themselves of the problem.

Misconceptions about hypnosis are widely prevalent in the general population, the commonest being that the person put in a trance relinquishes all controls, is completely under the control of the therapist or hypnotist, and therefore will be taken advantage of. Thus clients are often very apprehensive in the beginning, and it is very important that the therapist discusses their fears calmly, sympathetically and rationally. It is important never to laugh at a clients' fears or to ignore them. The therapist must also never argue with a client, because this will increase the client's defences and create resistance, and then the client will not respond as expected, leading to possible failure of the session. For similar reasons, the therapist should also not correct the client. It is often unnecessary to give detailed explanations about the nature of hypnosis, because this tends to become an intellectual exercise, and can sometimes be very boring for the patient. A variety of scientific scales have been devised to help clinicians in deciding whether a particular subject is likely to be easily hypnotised, called 'hypnotic susceptibility scales'. Some clinicians find these scales useful in clinical practice, but many others do not. Separate scales are available for children.

Research and clinical experience shows that in most people, trance can be induced quite rapidly, in a matter of a few minutes; therefore long-winded and elaborate induction techniques are a waste of time, can become quite boring for the client, and at worst, can increase the client's resistance. It is therefore important to match the pace of induction correctly while carefully observing the various physiological processes and changes that become apparent as the client enters the trance. These matters can only be learnt during training workshops.

When inducing a trance in a client, it is initially necessary to speak slowly, clearly and in a low tone. As the therapist gains confidence and feels more and more comfortable with the process of trance-induction, and also as the rapport with the patient increases over successive sessions, the therapist can begin to experiment with lowering the tone of voice even further, until it becomes almost inaudible. There is some clinical evidence that more effective trances can be obtained if the therapist speaks into the left ear of the client, rather than the right, because the left ear is neurologically connected to the right hemisphere of the brain, which is more concerned with functions such as visual imagery, musical awareness, dream-formation, creativity, emotions, spatial awareness, symbol formation, etc. – the 'holistic' aspects of functioning – whereas the left hemisphere is more concerned with functions such as mathematics, logic, reasoning, analysis, written language, reading and generally linear aspects of functioning. As we discussed earlier, the success of the hypnotic process largely depends upon direct communication with the unconscious mind, and the critical, conscious mind somewhat interferes with that process.

Hypnotherapy is an adjunctive treatment, which can be added to any other form of therapy. There are practically no contraindications for use of hypnosis; at worst, the hypnotic sessions may not cause any benefit. Even so, it is important to bear in mind that sometimes clients may present to the therapist when they are suffering from serious psychiatric conditions, such as schizophrenia, or severe depression, possibly with serious suicidal intent. Occasionally, the client's mental condition may arise from an underlying neurological condition, and in all these situations, it would be very prudent to make a cross-referral to a medically-qualified doctor, who may advise on the appropriateness, or otherwise, of using hypnotherapy.

A brief explanation of the three words 'hypnosis', 'hypnotherapy' and 'hypno-analysis' is in order. Hypnosis is the process of inducing trance. Hypnotherapy occurs when, after inducing the hypnotic trance, specific therapeutic suggestions are given to the client, with a view to reducing the client's symptoms or distress. Hypno-analysis is the process during which, after inducing hypnotic trance, techniques of psycho-analysis are used, such as free association, dream induction and dream analysis, automatic writing, hypnotic drawings, age regression to different ages and exploration of psychological resistances in the client.

Techniques of trance induction

There are three different methods of trance induction: the command method; the direct method (also sometimes called the standard relaxation method), and the indirect method (also called the Ericksonian or utilisation method). (The command method is used by stage hypnotists for entertainment purposes; it is *not* used by hypnotherapists.)

The direct or standard relaxation method

Lack of space prevents detailed description of the method for causing induction. However, interested readers are directed to authoritative texts, such as Waxman (1989).

This method requires the client to stare at a spot high up on a wall or the ceiling, and slow, elaborate suggestions are made that the eyes are watering . . . are getting tired . . . becoming heavy . . . and want to close, and that it is alright to close them when the subject wants to. There are numerous variations on this theme.

Signs of developing trance are as follows: if the eyes are open, gaze fixed with no blinking, eyes de-focused or immobile; if the eyes are closed, immobility of the body, a flat, 'ironed-out' look to the face, slow and deeper breathing, a slow pulse, sometimes the jaw sags and the mouth drops open, and the face often becomes paler than usual.

Increasingly, therapists are abandoning the authoritarian, direct approach in favour of more permissive and tolerant variations of the direct approach. An example of this is that rather than saying 'Now close your eyes', which would be authoritarian, the therapist might say 'When your eyes feel very heavy and they want to close, it is alright for you to close them.'

When the client closes their eyes, this is an indication that they have now entered a light trance. This should then be deepened, and some of the techniques of deepening are given below, while making careful observation about the client's respiration, eye movement, minor flickers in the muscles in the hands or fingers, and alterations in their heart rate, as evidenced by visible, peripheral pulsations, such as in the arteries in the neck. Furthermore, there are numerous guidelines and rules which, although they may appear quite trivial, are nevertheless very important in the successful and easy induction of trance as well as deepening, and therefore for the overall success of therapy. All this requires much practice, which can only be gained by joining teaching workshops.

The indirect or utilisation method

This was pioneered, and made extensive use of, by Milton Erickson (1901–1980), who was a hypnotherapist of extraordinary talent. He used very indirect methods of inducing trance, which placed emphasis on the interaction between the therapist and the subject, and he regularly used this approach to reduce or work around the resistances in the subject to being hypnotised.

The principle involved is as follows. The direct suggestion appeals to the conscious mind, and we respond by appropriate action. However, if the conscious mind was able to carry out all the suggestions, then it would be very easy for anyone to solve their problems, such as smoking or overeating. All those who are trying to give up smoking or to lose weight tell us how difficult they find it. Their conscious mind tells them to do it because it is rational; however, their unconscious mind causes impediments.

Recognising this, Erickson devised different ways of bypassing the negative influence of the unconscious mind, and designed suggestions which are so subtle that the unconscious mind does not recognise that a suggestion is being made. Rather than making prescriptive suggestions and therefore imposing control, as would happen with the direct method of induction, the indirect method emphasises interaction between the hypnotist and the client. The controls are given to the client, who decides whether to enter the trance, when to do so, and how deep to go, etc. This approach is therefore very much more flexible, underlining the fact that each client is an individual, and that the hypnotic suggestion must therefore adapt to this individuality.

Techniques of trance-deepening

Numerous methods are used for deepening the trance. In the 'arm levitation' method, a suggestion is made that as the client becomes more and more relaxed, one arm begins to feel lighter and lighter and gradually lifts off their lap or the chair on which it is resting, and as it lifts higher and higher, the subject goes deeper into trance. In the 'arm heaviness method', a suggestion is made that the arm which has been lifted high above the chair gradually begins to feel heavier and comes lower, finally to rest back in the subject's lap or on the arm of the chair, and as it comes down, the subject goes deeper and deeper into trance. In the 'counting up' method, a suggestion is made that as the therapist counts up from zero to say ten or twenty, the higher the count reaches, the deeper into trance the subject will go. A variation on this theme is 'counting down', where the reverse is suggested.

Another method is a 'guided walk' down a garden path, in which the subject is guided along an imaginary path down a very pleasant and beautiful garden, and the further they walk, the deeper they go into trance. A variation of this is to guide the subject down an imaginary flight of stairs, and as they climb down successive steps, they become more and more relaxed, and go deeper and deeper into trance.

A curious method sometimes used is where the therapist begins to count down from forty, but after reaching about the halfway mark, without previous instruction or forewarning, the count is reversed and the therapist begins to count upwards again. The confusion which is thus created has a unique effect and creates an intense and deep trance.

In the fractionation technique, the client is hypnotised, brought out of the trance to the state of full awakening, quickly hypnotised again, brought out of the trance again, and this process is repeated several times to achieve a very deep trance. Sometimes, when the subject has been hypnotised a few times by the same therapist, it is possible to use a short-cut method, in which the therapist may simply ask the client: 'Show me what you look like when you are in a deep trance.' More often than not, the client will oblige by going into a deep trance.

These are only some of the techniques for trance-deepening, but there are many more, and experienced therapists may be able to devise their own unique trance-deepening techniques.

Post-hypnotic suggestion

This means that the subject or client begins to act on a suggestion which has been given during the deep hypnotic trance only after they come out of the trance and are fully awake. In many ways, post-hypnotic suggestion forms the essence of a session of hypnotherapy, because clients come seeking help from the therapist about the problems that bother them during their waking hours, and therefore the solution ought to involve their actions during the waking hours.

An example of post-hypnotic suggestion is the therapist saying: 'When you hear me snap my fingers, you will at once close your eyes and go into a deep hypnotic sleep again.' Later, the client is brought out of the trance and woken up, and after a few minutes, the therapist may snap their fingers once or twice, upon which the client instantly passes into a deep hypnotic trance. The variations on this theme are numerous, with suggestions that the clients should do x, y or z when the therapist does a, b or c.

Very constructive use can be made of this very powerful method in altering the client's behaviour during waking hours. Post-hypnotic suggestions form the mainstay of a stage hypnotist's performance. However, in responsible sessions of hypnotherapy, amusing and embarrassing post-hypnotic suggestions must *not* be included.

Special considerations in hypnotherapy with children

One of the most important attributes of a therapist is that they should feel completely comfortable and confident in simply being with and interacting with children, and they should also have had considerable experience of working with children in different settings. Most authorities and clinicians agree that it is very easy to induce hypnotic trance in children. It is common knowledge that it is very natural for young children to talk to or play with imaginary friends, and indeed, this may be a form of self-hypnosis.

When practising hypnotherapy with children, considerable groundwork needs to be done, often more than with adult clients. It is necessary to consider who made the referral, and what the presenting problems are. It is often very useful to have some hypothesis about why a referral may have been made at this point. Emotional or behavioural problems in children almost always have their roots in factors of family dynamics and intrafamilial relationships; thus it is important to make some assessment about factors which are likely to influence the outcome of hypnotherapy, either positively or negatively. Such factors may include the motivation of the parents, secondary gains to the child from the symptoms, whether the child's behaviour is oppositional and wilful or the result of some important event in the family's lifecycle, etc. For these reasons, it is recommended that at least the first sessions should take place with the whole family wherever possible, and a full assessment of family dynamics should be carried out.

The clinician should then try to establish a good rapport with the child and try to gauge two specific aspects: (1) why does the child think they have been referred to the clinician, and what is their understanding of the problem; (2) what is the child's motivation in overcoming the problem. It is important to establish the child's attitude towards themself and their problems. If the child is quite pessimistic, then it is probably not a good idea to give the child a pep-talk by saying things like 'Oh, you will be alright,' because this is ego-dystonic for the child, and it interferes with establishing adequate rapport. In these circumstances, it is generally advisable that the therapist acknowledges and recognises the child's pessimism, and initially matches it, and then gradually tries to influence it in a positive direction by telling the child some stories about other children in similar circumstances whom the therapist might have seen in the past and who then improved.

Necessary theoretical background

Unlike adults, children's abilities vary enormously according to their age and stage of development. Of particular importance are the child's cognitive level, language development and emotional maturity. For example, a 2-year-old child cannot recall or remember, whereas a 3-year-old is able to do that; 4-year-old children understand sentences incorporating words such as 'because' and 'if', and have highly-developed fantasy and imagery. These factors will decide the types of induction methods to be used with children of different age groups. For this reason, it is imperative that the therapist has a good working and theoretical knowledge about child development, in particular the theories of cognitive development of Piaget, the psycho-analytic theories of development of mind and personality of Sigmund Freud, and the later neo-Freudian theories of Milton Erickson. The reader is advised to refer to other, more extensive texts on these matters; for example, Wall (1991) has considered these developmental issues in considerable detail.

It is uncertain whether a definite view can be held that children under 4 can be hypnotised in the same way as adults or children over the age of 12. The general principle would be that in very young children, communication needs to be non-verbal. For example, children up to 2 years of age are calmed (put in a trance) by rocking, patting, rhythmic singing, etc. For slightly older children, from the ages of 2 to 5, it is very useful to talk to them through the use of puppets; also, stories with 'because' causality and the word 'if' can be used very widely. From the age of 3 to about 10, fantasies and imagery can be used extensively. From the age of 5 to 12, children are amenable to the use of eye-closure techniques, and metaphors can also be used extensively. Some authorities suggest that a suggestion such as 'go to sleep' should not be used with young children, because it may frighten them; however, some other authorities do not necessarily find this an impediment. Along with this, techniques involving a 'special place', 'magic carpet', 'favourite sport' or 'favourite TV programme or favourite cartoon character' can also be used, as these are very effective. Above the age of 12, adult methods of trance induction, as described earlier, should be used.

Special scales for assessing children's hypnotic susceptibility are also available, but their usefulness is somewhat debatable. It is important to bear in mind that adult signs of hypnotic trance, such as physical relaxation, eye closure, etc., may not occur in very young children. Indeed, young children up to the age of about 6 are often frightened at the suggestion of closing their eyes, and in fact, they can be hypnotised with their eyes open. It is therefore very important that the therapist takes a very flexible and non-authoritarian approach to trance induction. Children have a very short attention span, which is partly determined by their developmental state and partly by the presenting psychopathology; therefore it is quite common for children, when they are in trance, to be quite fidgety, restless and even to open their eyes if they were shut during the trance, and to look around. This often baffles inexperienced therapists, but can easily be dealt with by the therapist saying something like: 'It is quite alright to open your eyes and to look around to make sure that everything is where it was when you closed your eyes first, and then when you are ready for it, you may close your eyes again.' Because children can be hypnotised very easily, it is often quite unnecessary to use a long and elaborate induction routine; in fact, this can be very boring for young children. With young children up to the age of 10 or 12, the hypnotic session should preferably not last longer than 20 minutes. Adult-style induction routines can be used for children aged 12 years and above, and the length of the hypnotic session can exceed 30 minutes.

Even though a child may not need any explanation of hypnosis, their parents often need it, and some demand it, because of their own preconceptions. When it comes to the induction of the hypnotic trance itself, there is no hard and fast rule about whether parents should be present or should be asked to leave the therapist's office. Most therapists feel that it is better to see the child on their own, because the parents might undermine or interfere with the process. On the other hand, it may be argued that if they are allowed to stay in the room, they will feel more reassured. I think, at the end of the day, this comes down to the therapist's own personal preference. Of course, in the case of younger children who may have difficulties in separating from the parents, their presence in the room may be advisable.

It is often a good idea to ask the child to practise self-hypnosis between sessions at home, as this will increase their sense of mastery and responsibility. Parental influence after the session also needs to be taken into consideration. If parents are overinvolved and enmeshed, and if it is the therapist's view that the child's difficulties are at least partly to do with this aspect of the parent–child relationship, then the parents should be counselled and advised that when the child practises self-hypnosis at home between sessions, they are to give the child the responsibility for it, and not to keep reminding the child or nagging them. If the child fails to practise, then the therapist will discuss it directly with the child. On the other hand, if the parents appear to be emotionally distanced from the child, then the parents' involvement and co-operation should be encouraged.

Special methods of induction for children

For children above the age of approximately 6 years, the method of eye-fixation and progressive relaxation described earlier can be used. A variation on this theme is that the child is requested to hold a reasonably heavy coin between the thumb and first finger, asked to raise the arm above the head and to stare at the thumbnail, with the suggestion that their eyes are watering, their eyelids are feeling heavy and want to close, and that the coin feels heavy, so that it will eventually drop. Reassurance can be given that the child need not worry about the coin, which can be picked up later; also, to encourage staring at the thumbnail, a little smiling face may be drawn on it with a felt-tip pen.

It is often better to ask the child to sit in a comfortable chair when inducing a trance, rather than asking them to lie down. Children usually have a greater tendency than adults to be unable to support their own body weight when in trance, and therefore often become like loosely-stuffed rag dolls. This tendency itself can be constructively used in inducing a trance – for example, the therapist might say 'Show me what you would look like if you were to become like a rag doll.'

Another technique is to ask the child about their favourite television programme, and to ask them to imagine that they are watching it. The child can then describe it, and the therapist can gradually enter the child's fantasy and use it to induce a trance. The same can be done by asking the child about their favourite cartoon character, and then manipulating the imagery. Other techniques, particularly for children aged 6–10, involve asking the child to imagine sitting on a magic carpet, on a magical journey, to describe their own favourite place or a favourite story. When encouraging such fantasy and imagination, the therapist may gently suggest that the child may, if they wish, close their eyes, because it is easier to see this special favourite place, the television programme, etc., when you close your eyes. In a sense, these are all ways of encouraging the child to enter a world of imagination and fantasy, with its own attendant altered state of awareness, which is hypnosis.

There are innumerable different ways of inducing a trance; the possibilities are limitless and really depend upon the therapist using their own initiative, spontaneity and creativity. (For descriptions of other techniques, the reader is directed to more detailed texts.)

Techniques of deepening the trance

There is some controversy about whether it is necessary to deepen the trance in children. If the therapist decides to do so, then many of the adult methods described earlier can be used. Fractionation is often a very useful and powerful method. Another is counting down from twenty to zero or ten to zero, while repeatedly suggesting that as the count goes down, the child becomes more and more relaxed. A variation on this is the suggestion of a downward movement, such as walking down the stairs of a very beautiful and colourful garden, and with each step that the child climbs down they become more and more relaxed. Another method is to ask the child to imagine that they are at a fairground ... holding a bunch of balloons, the strings tied to their first finger ... and with the breeze the balloon starts to lift up ... and up ... and with it lifts the child's finger ... and then their whole arm. Thus when arm levitation is achieved, it is coupled with the suggestion that as the arm lifts higher, the child becomes more and more relaxed. Later on, it may be suggested that the wind has dropped, and therefore the balloon gradually comes down, and with it, down comes the child's arm, and as the arm comes down, the child becomes more and more relaxed, and when the arm falls in their lap, they will be completely relaxed.

Making therapeutic suggestions

Of course, these will vary from child to child and from problem to problem. It is always a good idea to make a suggestion about increasing confidence in any hypnotic session. Also, as a guiding principle, it is generally considered that rather than making direct, authoritarian suggestions (such as 'From tomorrow, you will stop wetting your bed'), it is better to make a permissive suggestion (such as 'Perhaps one of these days you might find that you have stopped wetting the bed'). Authoritarian suggestions do often work; however, they can create a problem for the client, in that if the suggestion does not work, then the client will consider it as their total failure. Tilton (1987) describes a simple and excellent technique of using wires and switches. When analgesia is desired in a particular part of the body, the child is encouraged to imagine wires connected to that part and to find a switch, which is located somewhere else, which will turn that part on and off as desired.

Termination of trance

This is usually quite a simple procedure. The therapist might count down from ten to zero, repeatedly suggesting that as they count, the child is becoming more and more aware of their surroundings and alert, and at the count of zero, will wake up and open their eyes, feeling very refreshed. If the induction technique had involved imagining watching the television, then the therapist might simply suggest that the child switches the television off. Generally speaking, the termination should be complementary to the induction routine.

Treatment of anxiety by hypnosis in children

Anxiety can be both cause and effect. When anxiety is the cause, it can manifest itself in production of symptoms such as tics, school refusal, different phobias, disorders of sleep such as nightmares, and disorders of sleep cycle (such as inability to fall asleep or waking up at unusual times), different phobias, and somatisation disorders affecting different systems – these would include enuresis, soiling, asthma, eczema, nausea or vomiting. In addition, there may be generalised anxiety disorder, with anxiety being the trait. When anxiety is the effect, the basic cause may be situations such as: a general lack of confidence (trait anxiety); anxiety arising out of trauma, such as bullying at school, physical or sexual abuse, witnessing of violence at home (such as violence in parental marriage); post-traumatic stress disorder caused by a traumatic event; pain such as that arising out of a terminal illness (cancer); conditions like leukaemia, where painful procedures such as bone marrow transplant are required, or pain from surgical procedures, burns, etc.

In all these conditions in children (and many more), hypnotherapy can be used, often with excellent results, in order to alleviate the symptoms and cause relief. As mentioned earlier, when treating any child, it is strongly advisable to initially meet with the whole family wherever possible, to make a full assessment of the family dynamics and factors, strengths and weaknesses which might aid or interfere with treatment.

Generalised anxiety

This sometimes develops because the child is unable to share with other significant adults around them (such as parents, other family members, teachers, etc.) the real source of their worry. What others see, therefore, is an anxious child, without understanding the source of the anxiety. After inducing the trance and making the child relax deeply, the child is encouraged to talk about their fears, problems and sources of worries. This should be done in a gentle manner, in such a way that the child will not be overwhelmed. Specific suggestions can be given to increase their confidence about their worth and capability, thus generally strengthening their ego. Another useful suggestion to make is that the child may model themselves on their favourite hero (which information will have been gathered during the interview before induction of hypnotic trance), emphasising the qualities that the child finds appealing in this hero. They can also be encouraged to use self-hypnosis at home.

School refusal and phobia

It is necessary to determine the reasons behind the school-based anxiety which presents as school refusal or phobia. Some common reasons behind this anxiety are: being physically bullied; having an awkward teacher that the child cannot get on with; intellectual difficulties with problems of understanding the coursework, and the resultant fear that the child might make a fool of themselves, or worries about the physical health of a significant family member, usually the mother. After understanding the reason, appropriate suggestions can be made under the hypnotic trance – for example, if bullying is the worry, then the suggestions would be about increasing self-confidence, strengthening the ego, and a positive suggestion that they will find themselves becoming physically and emotionally stronger, and quite soon will be able to stand their ground, and deal with people who do not always co-operate with them. Other underlying causes will attract other suitable suggestions.

Tics

Deep relaxation should be induced, with positive suggestion that the child is in full control of their body and its movements, and no tics can develop if they decide that they should not.

Phobias

Phobias are often conditioned responses – for example, a dog snarls and growls fiercely and barks loudly at a child, then the child becomes phobic of dogs. The treatment can lie in carrying out desensitisation procedures under a deep hypnotic trance. In addition, ego-strengthening suggestions, and suggestions for increased confidence, should always be given.

Obsessive and compulsive features

Here also, relaxation and desensitisation can be used.

Sleep problems

In a child who used to sleep well before, it is important to establish the causality for the onset of sleep disturbance. Some common reasons for anxiety related to sleep are: impending breakdown of stable family relationships, such as parental divorce; witnessing violence, usually intra-familial, such as father's violence towards the mother; watching violent videos which are unsuitable for the child's age; significant traumatic events involving the family, such as burglary, fire at home, etc., and significant school problems, such as severe bullying and child sexual abuse. Having discovered the real source of anxiety, it should be tackled in an appropriate manner. Child sexual abuse must be reported to the child protection team of the local authority. Trance-deepening techniques are very useful. A post-hypnotic suggestion can be that every night, when the child puts their head on the pillow to go to sleep, they will fall asleep. It is always advisable to ask the child to practise self-hypnosis at home.

Enuresis

Like sleep, in a child who was previously dry at night, onset of bed-wetting needs to be investigated carefully. The causes for this are generally the same as those which cause sleep disturbance, discussed above. After determining the source of anxiety, the appropriate course of action should be taken. Many methods of treatment of enuresis are available, and these include star charts, bell and pad (also called 'pad and buzzer'), bladder retraining, use of medication, etc. This is possibly the only clinical condition which may be treated with the child lying down on a couch. Hypnotic suggestion should be commensurate with the nature of the source of anxiety. Suggestions for increasing confidence and ego-strengthening should also be given. Another specific suggestion can be that the child is strong and intelligent, and only they will control all the functions of their body (implying that their bladder will not contract, causing bedwetting, if they do not want that to happen). Yet another way of doing this is to make the child aware and sensitive of perceiving the fullness of the bladder while still under hypnotic trance, then to suggest that they may get up from the bed, open their eyes, go to the nearest toilet, urinate, return to the therapist's room, lie down on the couch and immediately fall into a deep sleep. When these actions are carried out, and the child enters trance again, a post-hypnotic suggestion will be given that when they return home and sleep in their own bed, they will become aware when their bladder fills up; they will then get out of bed, go to the toilet, empty their bladder and return to bed. In the morning, they will find a dry bed. It is better to make permissive suggestions, rather than authoritarian ones, for reasons already mentioned.

Somatisation disorders

Respiratory system: Asthma

This is also often related to anxiety. The source of that anxiety should be uncovered and dealt with appropriately. Hypnotic suggestions should also be appropriate to the source; thus if the anxiety is school-based and related to bullying, then proceed as outlined above.

Gastro-intestinal system

Tummy aches In children, tummy ache on a school morning is very common, and is related to school anxiety; therefore it should be investigated appropriately and treated as outlined above.

Nausea and vomiting These two, along with tummy ache on school mornings, complete a picture of school-related anxiety, and therefore should be treated along the same lines as school refusal, mentioned above. Sometimes, nausea and vomiting are related to intake of cytotoxic drugs, such as those given to treat cancer and leukaemia. In these situations, the nausea and vomiting is often a conditioned response, and can be usefully treated by inducing a deep trance and giving a positive suggestion. Regular self-hypnosis at home is extremely useful.

Soiling This is often treated by doctors through the use of medication, stool-softeners, enemas, dietary advice including a high-fibre diet, and occasionally admission to a ward for bowel retraining. When the soiling is the result of constipation with overflow, the problem is often that the lower bowel (large intestine) is so grossly dilated that it loses the sensation of distension, which in normal people would cause a natural reflex to defecate. In these circumstances, under the hypnotic trance, the child is asked to pay careful attention to the sensation in their tummy, and when they are aware of the 'blown-up' feeling, they should then go to the toilet and defecate. This increase in the sensitivity to the state of the bowel is often quite crucial in the treatment of soiling with hypnotherapy. In addition, another suggestion to make is that the child is a strong and intelligent person, and they alone can control their body functions.

Skin problems

Eczema and atopic dermatitis ('nervous eczema') are often related to asthma, and the underlying psychopathology is often suppressed anger. It is most important to reassure the child that their skin condition is not contagious. Hypnotic suggestions involve increase in confidence and self-worth, ego-strengthening, and specific suggestions under deep trance, to encourage a feeling of cold, calm and smooth skin. Repeated self-hypnosis at home is strongly indicated. Kuttner (1991) mentions a case of a 4-year-old child with eczema where hypnotic trance was achieved with eyes open, and suggestions made to 'take this lovely soft cloud, scoop it up, and put it on the itchy parts, so that it makes your skin feel so good, soft, smooth and very calm'.

Management of pain

Pain arising from a terminal illness or medical procedures such as bone marrow transplantation, as required in the treatment of leukemia, can be very effectively treated with hypnotherapy. Under deep hypnotic trance, positive suggestions can be made that the child will feel brave when facing the pain, and it will hurt less. It is often very useful to ask the child's opinion about what needs to change so that the pain will hurt less. The child might, for example, say that the injection would hurt less if their arm were made of wood, or if their body were covered with metal armour. Such ideas from the child can then be incorporated during a deep hypnotic trance. Repeated self-hypnosis at home always enhances the desired effect.

Post-traumatic stress disorder and traumatic memories

When dealing with these conditions, in addition to the usual induction of deep trance, suggestion of deep relaxation and ego-strengthening, suggestions are made about reduction in the experienced symptoms. Another technique involves making use of the primary sensory modalities (visual, auditory and kinaesthetic); however, this technique is much more specific, cannot be described in words, and really needs to be learnt in a professional skill-development workshop.

Sexual abuse and rape

Use of hypnotherapy for treatment of these two situations is an extremely skilled job. It must be remembered that being in a one-to-one situation with the therapist, especially if it happens to be a male therapist, in the therapist's office with the door closed, and if the therapist suggests eye closure as part of the induction routine, is very reminiscent of the situation in the child's life where sexual abuse or rape originally occurred. It is therefore not surprising that under such circumstances, the child will resist working with the therapist, and for these reasons, such work must only be carried out by extremely skilled therapists.

Final comment

In the recent past, the media have given much publicity to a condition called 'false memory syndrome', in which patients in therapy which had taken place many years ago accused the significant other adults in their lives of abusing them; these other adults, in return, accused the therapists of implanting memories in their patients of events that did not actually occur. Hypnotherapy would appear to be particularly vulnerable to such accusations, because of the very nature of induction of trance, and also the mysticism which surrounds it among the general public. Hypnotherapists therefore need to take great precautions to avoid such allegations being made against them. It may be a good idea to videotape the session, wherever such facilities are available. It must also be remembered that a hypnotherapy session which occurs behind closed doors in the therapist's office, with the client's eyes closed and the client in a state of a deep relaxation, is also a very intense one-to-one situation, which leaves both the client and the therapist potentially very vulnerable. It is therefore most important that the therapist observes a strict professional attitude and completely respects their client's individuality as well as confidentiality.

Conclusion

In this chapter, an attempt has been made to describe the basics of the theory and practice of hypnotherapy. This is by no means a comprehensive account of this very fascinating field. If the reader feels stimulated to read more exhaustive and authoritative texts or seek training, then the purpose of this chapter has been served.

References

Ambrose, G. (1961) *Hypnotherapy with Children* (2nd edn), London: Staples.
Breuer, J. & Freud, S. (1955) 'Studies on hysteria', in Strachey, J. (ed.) *The Standard Edition of the Complete Psychological Works of Sigmund Freud*, Vol.II: 1893–1895, London: Hogarth Press, pp.21–47.

Erickson, M.H. (1964) 'The confusion technique in hypnosis', *American Journal of Clinical Hypnosis*, 6, pp.183–207.

Haley, J. (1986) *Uncommon Therapy*, New York: W.W. Norton.

Kuttner, L. (1991) 'Special considerations for using hypnosis with young children', in Wester, W.C. II and O'Grady, D.J. (eds) *Clinical Hypnosis with Children*, New York: Brunner/Mazel.

O'Hanlon, W.H. & Hexum, A.L. (1990) *An Uncommon Casebook: Complete Clinical Work of Milton H. Erickson*, New York: W.W. Norton.

Shor, R.E. (1969) 'Hypnosis and the concept of the generalised reality orientation', in Tart, P. (ed.) *Altered States of Consciousness*, New York: Anchor-Doubleday.

Tilton, P. (1987) 'Hypnotic techniques with children', in Schaefer, C.E. (ed.) *Innovative Interventions in Child Adolescent Therapy*, New York: John Wiley, p.144.

Wall, V. (1991) 'Developmental considerations in the use of hypnosis with children', in Wester, W.C. II and O'Grady, D.J. (eds) *Clinical Hypnosis with Children*, New York: Brunner/Mazel.

Waxman, D. (1989) *Hartland's Medical and Dental Hypnosis* (3rd edn), London: Baillière Tindall, p.6.

Wester, W.C. II and O'Grady, D.J. (1991) *Clinical Hypnosis with Children*, New York: Brunner/Mazel, p.xvi.

13 Cultural aspects of anxiety in children

Vaman Lokare

Introduction

Since World War II, there has been increasing interest in cross-cultural problems. The reason for this is obviously multifactorial. Perhaps one of the reasons is the situation where the individual has difficulty forming and maintaining identity, which is nowadays to be seen in many European countries with 'guest workers', and in Britain with settlers from Commonwealth countries who form minority groups. Even countries like the USA and the Netherlands are not free of problems of cultural identity, with its attendant anxieties and consequences (Essed, 1991).

Members of minority cultural identity groups often identify themselves with the dominant majority, and in their attempts to assimilate in the dominant culture, they sometimes change their names or religion, and try actively to reject and forget their old customs, language and lifestyle, etc. Individuals may be seen to vacillate between two cultures. Many who had lived in some degree of isolation before, due to better communications, have increased contact, as in the case of the Inuit and Lapps (Forsius, 1975). This struggle with identity often creates feelings of insecurity, leading to anxieties and worries which are reflected as feelings of uncertainty and insufficiency in bringing up one's own children and giving them rules, norms and traditions to follow. Often, this kind of struggle to attain cultural identity becomes enmeshed with ethnic identity and problems of racial discrimination.

The concept of 'culture' causes difficulties, as the word is often confused with the word 'race'. Both these words are emotionally charged, as people associate them with acts of discrimination. A useful way of understanding these concepts could be to follow the first statement on race issued by UNESCO:

199

a group or population characterised by some concentrations, relative as to frequency and distribution, or hereditary particles (genes) or physical characters which appear, fluctuate and often disappear in the course of time by reason of geographic and/or cultural isolation. (Montague, 1972, p.7)

Anthropologists' classification of humans never includes mental characteristics. Race can also be understood as subgroups of people with similar habits, customs, sentiments and attitudes.

It is clear from this that differences between races are also related to social and environmental variables, and this makes real study of racial psychological differences almost impossible. Culture therefore comes very much to the fore when the question is raised of what is associated with the socio-economic adjustment, frustrations and conflicts, anxiety and stress in different nations and communities, and in particular in a multicultural and multinational setting.

Understanding culture and anxiety

The human child is born into a society which is made up of a group of people dependent upon one another, who have developed patterns of behaviour essential for survival and growth of the group. Even among primitive peoples, group association was recognised to have value for both the individual and the group. An infant (and older child) depends upon others for the satisfaction of needs. The ways in which these others meet these needs, and the infant's (and older child's) responses to their behaviour, become fundamental factors of social development. Hence it is important for every child to learn the ready-made pattern of behaviour and thinking that exists in society and which is transmitted from generation to generation within a continuing society, as this is essential for the individual's survival as the society develops.

These prescribed patterns of behaviour, customs, beliefs, etc., make up a large aspect of what is meant by 'culture'. As McKeachie and Doyle (1966) put it: 'we consider culture to be the patterns of behaving and thinking and products of behaviour that are transferred from generation to generation within any continuing society'. So growth and development are closely linked with the physical, mental and emotional aspects of development. The child is therefore at the mercy of numerous factors in the cultural, social, economic and natural environment, and is continually being changed or moulded by the surrounding world, and the child's progress in the world is therefore filled with success, failure, frustration, stress and anxiety.

The behaviour and attitudes of an individual are regarded as normal or abnormal according to the cultural milieu in which the behaviour takes place. However, most societies are not rigid taskmasters, and allow reasonable latitude for individuality of expression. Radical aberrations that create turmoil in individuals or those around them are usually looked upon as abnormal behaviour and/or evidence of abnormal personality. Horney (1937) described anxiety as a feeling of hopelessness in a potentially hostile world. This, according to her, develops out of interplay between feelings of anxiety and hostility stirred up by rejecting parental attitudes, and is the cause of neurosis. She suggests that many reactions which we look upon as being neurotic in one culture are considered quite normal in another, and also that many conflicts developed by the individual mirror the contradictions in their society.

Mead (1953) says that 'culture':

> is the term applied to the total shared learning behaviour of a society or a subgroup so we may speak of 'a culture', using the term for a whole, or for an item of behaviour as 'cultural', as referring this item to the whole. The moral situation on which the anthropological aspect of culture is based, is that of the total learned, shared behaviour of a functional autonomous society that has maintained its existence through a sufficient number of generations, so that each stage of the life span of the individual is included within the system. (pp.57–82)

Gorer (1953) extends this to mean that culture is:

> primarily mental or physiological, as non-biological learned behaviour ultimately derivable from the nerves and brain cells of the personnel comprising a given society at a given time.

He also says:

> cultural behaviour is learned behaviour ... learning can be divided into two categories: (1) learning situations in which certainly the teacher, and usually the pupil are conscious and can be articulate about what is being taught, and (2) learning that is not articulate or verbalised by the teacher (if there is one) may not be conscious of teaching and which may not be imparted or deliberately conceptualised as a total concept.

In fact, he sees culture as the result of both kinds of learning.

The term 'culture' in this chapter refers to more or less organised and relatively persistent patterns of habits, ideas, attitudes, bodies of knowledge, skills and values in a society which are passed on to individuals, and which, to a large extent, individuals imitate, intentionally or unintentionally, as this provides them with the framework within which they learn to function with those who are close to them. Therefore, one of the child's major responsibilities is to learn to adjust to the group or groups of which the child is a member. Depending on the ease or difficulty with which success is achieved in adjustment or failure, anxiety may be aroused. In other words, culture could, in some respects, be considered responsible for anxiety. Change may take place over centuries, or even within a decade. For Sinha (1962), culture is basic to anxiety. This raises the question: what is anxiety, and how do we define it?

Anxiety is a universal experience. It has been described as a form of vigilance which occurs after encountering danger. McDougall (1908) says that anxiety is a complex emotion, and is essentially a matter of alertness or watchfulness. According to Freud (1955), a child inherits the 'tendency towards objective anxiety'. Freud also believed that objective anxiety is an expression of the self-preservation instinct, and has obvious utility as a defence. Freud's 'objective anxiety' involves traumatic factors, and he talks of primary and secondary objective anxiety. Traumatic factors such as the birth trauma are involved in the occurrence of primary objective anxiety, while secondary objective anxiety is elicited by the likelihood of occurrence of a traumatic event. Judging from the accounts by Hoch and Zubin (1950), Rosenberg (1949) and Roycroft (1968), this seems to be the current psycho-analytic position. Still remaining within the psycho-analytical realm, anxiety may be conceived as a:

> conscious danger signal associated, not only with an external danger, but also with unconscious contents and motivations, the conscious elaboration of which is inhibited or defended against, because such elaboration would place the individual in even more dangers in relation to the external world. (Sarason et al., 1960)

Drever (1958) defines anxiety as:

> a chronic, complex emotional state with apprehension or dread as its most prominent component characteristics of various nervous and mental disorders.

Anxiety is defined by May (1950) as:

> the apprehension cued off by a threat to some value which the individual holds essential to his existence as a personality.

Anxiety could also be defined as an innate capacity of an organism to react, and it has some inherited neurophysiological concomitants:

> the particular forms which this capacity to react to threats will assume in a given individual is conditioned by the nature of the threats (environment) and by how the individual has learned to deal with them (past and present experience). (May, 1950)

This definition suggests that there is a strong influence from upbringing, social and cultural learning on anxieties in an individual.

In recent years, psychologists have attempted to relate the concept of anxiety to learning theories. Both learning theorists and psycho-analysts reflect a somewhat deterministic view of behaviour, as they deal with plans and goals as products of experimental histories in individuals. However, while psycho-analysis is preoccupied with the explanation of deviant behaviour and makes no clear-cut distinction between maturation and socialisation as a matter of learning, learning theorists emphasise carefully-controlled experiments to test specific hypotheses about how socialisation influences personality, and they apply the results of such experiments to the area of psychopathology.

Mowrer's view of anxiety almost makes the need for experiments to explain psychopathology unnecessary. Mowrer (1950) says that anxiety comes not from the individual's 'acts which he has committed but wishes he had not. It is, in other words, a guilt theory of anxiety rather than an impulse theory'. Mowrer also thinks that the only difference between Pavlov and Freud is that the former thought that the danger signal (conditioned stimulus) elicits the same reaction that was previously produced by actual trauma (stimulus substitution), whereas the latter thought that a danger signal may produce any one of the infinite variety of possible reactions that are unlike those reactions to the original trauma. In other words, this is recasting Freud's theory of anxiety into a stimulus-response (SR) terminology. It was this that led Mowrer (1939) to assume a theory of fear as a drive, and fear reduction as reinforcement, which he later tested. He found that anxiety reduction was positively correlated with learning.

Miller and Dollard (1941) talk of anxiety in terms of its drive properties, and believe that anxiety is one of the major sources of human motivation. They think drive is innate, and what is acquired is the tendency for a previously neutral stimulus to elicit the drive. In fact, it is the association between the stimulus and drive that has been acquired.

To test these hypotheses derived from learning theory, Taylor (1956) starts from Hull's (1943) basic assumption that the excitatory potential E, determining the strength of a response, is a multiplicative function of a learning factor H and a generalised drive factor D, so that $E = H \times D$. He assumes that the drive level D is the function of the magnitude or strength of a hypothetical response in the organism – persistent emotional response in the organism which he calls r (fear or anxiety) – and conceives drive due to anxiety as non-specific. A similar approach has also been used by Castaneda et al. (1956) in their work with the Children's Manifest Anxiety Scale.

Sarason and Mandler (1952) view anxiety as being situation-specific, and aroused in an achievement situation. This they call 'test anxiety'. They emphasise anxiety as drive stimulus (SD). This can be interpreted to mean that 'anxiety reactions are generalised from previous experience to the testing situation' (Miller & Dollard, 1941, cited in Sarason & Mandler, 1952).

If anxiety is given this status of a drive, then in terms of the Yerkes-Dodson principle (1908), it would seem to follow Pavlov's laws: the law of strength and the law of transmarginal inhibition. The former asserts that the response strength is proportional to the strength of the stimulus, and the latter that there is a point of maximum response beyond which any further increase in strength of the stimulus leads to a lessening of response.

In terms of the Yerkes-Dodson principle, the relationship between a drive and learning is curvilinear, and is referred to as the 'inverted-U relation between drive and performance'. There is an optimal level of drive for each kind of task, which energises the individual and helps to improve performance. While too low a drive, below optimal level, may produce insufficient motivation, and may be inadequate to improve performance, too high a level of drive that exceeds the optimal for a given task may interfere with the learning processes and prove to be disruptive, and may even lead to maladaptive responses (Lokare, 1966, 1972a, 1972b). Furthermore, one also has to consider seriously the results of applying the second half of the Yerkes-Dodson principle, which says that the relationship between drive and performance is a function of task complexity, in that for very simple tasks, the optimal level is high, while very difficult tasks have a low optimal drive level. It would therefore follow that the drive level that facilitates performance on a simple task may disrupt it when the task is more complex and difficult.

If we add to these suggestions the fact that a heightened drive state (anxiety) is linked with a number of previously-learned response tendencies, often emotional in nature and even irrelevant to the task in hand, and which disrupt performance by competing with the right response (Sarason & Mandler, 1952; Child, 1954), then we reach a situation well described by Jones (1960):

> When the correct response is based on relatively weak habit strength, increased drive is deleterious in that the stronger inaccurate tendencies gain relatively more in excitatory potential, and have therefore an enhanced probability of evocation. (pp.488–528)

Here we can add one more controversial but widely-used definition of anxiety, labelled as emotionality, neuroticism or instability, which is one part of a two-dimensional system of personality description (Eysenck, 1970), and which claims to have strong hereditary biases and yet interlocks with certain social and psychiatric methods of classification (Eysenck, 1967).

If culture is related to anxiety, and anxiety is related to the concept of learning theories, it should be obvious that the number of possible definitions of anxiety may be unlimited; but by now, it should be obvious that all take their origins from some theoretical orientation, and hence, to a certain extent, have abstract contents that often fulfil operational criteria. However, all these definitions could be classed under either one or both of these classifications: (1) habitual, innate or trait-anxiety, with possible hereditary bias, and (2) situation-produced anxiety in undifferentiated groups of subjects.

The definitions that fall strictly within the first classification emphasise the hereditary nature of anxiety, and imply a possible (so-called) racial difference in anxiety. The definitions that fall totally within the second classification suggest strong cultural and subcultural limitations, and expose anxiety to the total mercy of environmental effects in terms of upbringing and education.

A modern-day psychologist therefore considers anxiety as a complex concept with respect to its origin, its behavioural effects and its interindividual differences. It is generally accompanied by some psychosomatic changes, for example increase in perspiration, heart rate, etc. While anxiety in accord with reality could be considered essential, and even beneficial, disproportionate anxiety could be a handicap, and may even lead to psychopathological conditions.

Differences in anxiety in girls and boys

Research over the last few decades shows, unequivocally, that girls score higher than boys on all the anxiety scales, irrespective of the theoretical orientation on which the tests are constructed. One could interpret this to mean that girls are more anxious than boys, that they feel anxiety in a wider variety of situations, and that they also feel it more intensively than boys.

One could say that the reason for the marked differences in anxiety scores between girls and boys is due to the fact that it is easier for girls to admit to anxiety. This means that the differences in the anxiety scores between girls and boys do not reflect an innate difference, but are only a measure of differences in their attitude to admitting to anxiety. Kapoor (1964) suggests that the observed sex differences in psychological characteristics are mainly traceable to environmental factors, rather than any innate tendencies that are sex-linked. Talking of environmental and cultural factors makes boys more defensive in admitting anxiety, because in the cultures under study, they are supposed to be brave. Sarason's own alternative explanation as to why boys are more defensive in admitting anxiety implies that the answer may lie in the contents of the General Anxiety Scale for Children (GASC) itself, as it refers to fears and bodily injuries, etc., which he says boys are naturally likely to be less willing to admit. However, Lokare (1989) reports differences between girls and boys, but no significant differences in scores on the neuroticism scale on Lokare's Modified Junior Maudsley Personality Inventory (LMJMPI) for English, white, non-white and Indian children. This makes it difficult to accept explanations based purely on environmental and cultural considerations.

On the basis of this, one could easily make the mistake of jumping to the conclusion that anxiety is totally sex-linked, and in that sense, genetically determined. However, this would make it difficult to find an acceptable explanation for the differences found between the anxiety scores of girls on the GASC and TASC (Test Anxiety Scale for Children) reported by Sarason et al. (1960), Pringle and Cox (1963) and Nijhawan (1972), those found on the CMAS (Children's Manifest Anxiety Scale) by Levitt (1957), Palermo (1959), Rie (1963) and Colman et al. (1972) among Indian, white English, English non-white, white and black American girls, and differences between the scores of boys belonging to these various groups. Any attempt to find a purely hereditary explanation of anxiety and to attribute these differences in scores to racial differences would create further complications and lead to possible misunderstandings.

Sarason et al. (1960) report lower mean scores on the GASC for anxious English children than for white American children, although not significantly so. This differs significantly from the findings of Pringle and Cox (1963) for English children, and also those reported by Nijhawan (1972) for Indian children.

Sarason et al. (1960) also report significantly lower mean scores on the TASC for white American children than for the white English children. Pringle and Cox (1963) report similar findings. Nijhawan (1972) reports significantly higher mean scores on the TASC for Indian children than for both the American white and English white children.

The reports of mean scores on the CMAS vary widely from one researcher to another. Mean scores on the CMAS reported by Levitt (1957), Palermo (1959) and Rie (1963) show differences even between groups of white American children. Again, the scores on the CMAS for English children reported by Colman et al. (1972) and for black American children reported by Palermo (1959) are both significantly higher than those reported by Levitt (1957) for American white children. However, they do not differ significantly from those reported by Rie (1963) and Palermo (1959). It looks as though the mean scores, depending on the particular sample, may overlap across various racial and cultural groups, and may also differ significantly between samples from the same racial/cultural group.

In the LMJMPI scores, where anxiety is defined in terms of neuroticism, there is no significant difference in the reported scores for the children belonging to various samples, and this holds good regardless of their membership of any racial or cultural group.

One is tempted at this stage to assign the differences in anxiety scores to a complex and peculiar combination of differences in race, culture, education and upbringing. But one has to bear in mind the possibility that the differences in the anxiety scores could be chance differences, due to sampling error or the size of the samples being too small to test the hypothesis. It could also reflect the rigidity or the inadequacy of the theoretical orientation and the structure of each of these tests. Once again, among the reports on the GASC, TASC, CMAS and LMJMPI (Lokare, 1966, 1972a, 1972b and 1989), Lokare (1989) fails to show significant differences in the scores of children belonging to different racial and cultural groups. As mentioned earlier, this test defines anxiety in terms of neuroticism. The findings therefore strongly suggest that there are no racial or cultural differences in anxiety level in schoolchildren, and also that, possibly, the test measures a particular aspect or a special feature of anxiety which is uniformly distributed among all the members of the human race. It would also appear that this aspect is only insignificantly influenced by differences in culture, education or upbringing. This is borne out by Eysenck's (1959) studies with adults, where he reports no significant differences in the neuroticism scores for various samples of the American as well as the English population.

Age variations

The literature is full of studies which report age differences in anxiety. According to psycho-analytical and learning-theory approaches, from the time children start appraising their relationship with their parents and begin to react to the impact of evaluative quality of their behaviour, they should show an upward trend in the development of anxiety. Sarason (1959) and Thompson (1965), in their studies of the TASC, reported that anxiety increases with age. Eysenck (1965) reported a similar trend, in that girls become more unstable with increasing age, but this applies to boys of only 7 or 8 years of age. Lokare (1972b) also reported similar trends, but only in boys of 8, 9 and 10 years of age. In general, this would support Freud's theory, according to which, as the ego matures, there is an increase in the ability to judge events and to anticipate the future. With this comes a more realistic perception of danger, and consequently, an increase in anxiety. This would also support the theory that anxiety is learned and not inherited.

Therefore, it would seem to follow that to look for racial differences in anxiety would not be a rewarding exercise, as whatever differences are found could all have a strong cultural and educational stamp, in terms of learnt behaviour. However, Nijhawan (1972), in a study of the GASC and TASC, and Angelino et al. (1956), in their study of situation anxiety, reported that anxiety is somewhat negatively related to age. In their studies of the CMAS, both Palermo (1959) and Colman et al. (1972) reported that there is some indication of inverse relationship between age and anxiety. Eysenck (1965) reported a similar trend in boys aged 9 years upwards in her studies of the Junior Eysenck Personality Inventory. Lokare (1972b) also reported a similar trend in boys from 10 years upwards and girls from 8 years upwards. This suggests a possible strong influence of developmental factors related to maturation and growth in terms of psychophysiological mechanisms, rather than purely in terms of maturation of the ego or solely as the result of learning in terms of learning theories.

Besides, there is evidence to suggest that the basic tendency to react with anxiety diminishes, though only slightly, with very large increases in age, even in adults (Eysenck, 1970). All this implies that anxiety is a complex concept.

Socio-economic influence

The role played by socio-economic level in the emotional adjustment of the individual is still little understood. Opinions differ among authors on the issue of the relationship between socio-economic status and anxiety. Brown (1934) states that neuroticism does not predominate in any social or cultural group. However, in his later study (Brown, 1936), he reports that differences in emotional stability are not a function of either race or locale, but are closely related to socio-economic level. Springer (1938), using Brown's Personality Inventory for Children, the Haggarty and Oslon-Wickman Behaviour Rating Schedule, which is closely related to the general social status of the individual, and the Barr Scale of Occupational Status of Fathers, also arrived at the conclusion that emotional stability is closely related to the status of the individual child. Sarason et al. (1960) found that Milford children from lower socio-economic status families scored higher than Greenwich children belonging to upper-class families. Heywood and Dobbs (1964) reported that children from low socio-economic status groups scored higher on the CMAS than children from high socio-economic status groups. Durrett (1965), in his study on an Indian sample of Marathi-speaking children, reported a tendency for middle-class, middle-income children to score higher on the CMAS than children belonging to lower-income families, though the differences were not significant. Nijhawan (1972), in her study of Indian children, reported that the children of lower socio-economic class exhibited significantly higher anxiety than upper-class children on both the GASC and the TASC. There is a striking similarity between some of her results for upper-class Indian children and those figures for Western children reported by various authors.

At this stage, on still further reflection, some seemingly obvious explanations for the differences in anxiety scores come to mind. In addition to the racial and cultural differences between the various groups of children, there are also differences in their socio-economic status, which could be responsible for the differences. Two of the many studies on adults that support this view are those of Dahlstrom and Welsh (1960) on an American sample, and Joshi and Singh (1966) on an Indian sample. These findings add a further complication to the already complex problem of meaningful interpretation of differences in anxiety found between various groups of children, and even groups of adults, for that matter, belonging to different racial groups, minorities and nationalities. It makes the task of even planning comparative studies of racial and cultural differences much more difficult, as it is not easy to find comparable racial and cultural groups without any differences in their socio-economic level and social status. Besides, it would be difficult to estimate the amount of influence exerted on the level of anxiety by socio-economic level and social status, as these are, in turn, so interdependent with the cultural values and the philosophy of the people who make up the group.

Anxiety, education and achievements

So far, the whole of the discussion on anxiety has centred around group similarities and differences. It is time we looked at this in terms of individual differences. Fortunately, there seems to be universal agreement, irrespective of theoretical background and beliefs, that individuals differ to varying degrees. There is also agreement that children can be classified as showing high, low or intermediate levels of anxiety, and that in any given cross-section of society, the majority always belong to the group which shows neither particularly high nor low anxiety, irrespective of race or culture.

The effects of anxiety as a drive on behaviour have been assessed by studies of experimentally-induced anxiety, or by using children who have been found to exhibit high or low anxiety. Two important issues studied in this way are the relationship of anxiety in educational achievement, and the relationship of anxiety to behavioural adjustment. Sarason et al. (1960) reported significant negative correlations between anxiety and performance on educational achievement and intelligence tests. Gaudry and Bradshaw (1970) found that children with high anxiety score significantly lower in class tests than those with low anxiety. Cox (1960) also studied the relationship between anxiety and school assessment marks. He reported that about three-quarters of the medium-anxiety group were in the top half of the class, compared with approximately half of the low-anxiety group and less than one-third of the high-anxiety group. This seems to support Hebb's (1958) theory that optimal level of motivation for effective performance lies in the middle ranges, rather than at the high or low end. One can see how this also supports the formalised Yerkes-Dodson law (Yerkes & Dodson, 1908), which states that the relationship between motivation (anxiety) and learning takes the form of the inverted U-shaped curve mentioned earlier.

A vast number of studies carried out along these lines so far show that anxiety tends to impair children's problem-solving ability. The most consistent general findings so far are that high anxiety is associated with relatively low performance at both school and university level. This is irrespective of the type of test used for measuring anxiety and the varieties of measures of academic achievements used. Studies so far have also indicated that high-anxious children have more difficulty with complex learning tasks than low-anxious children, because of the arousal of competing responses, more of which are raised to threshold level for the high-anxious child. However, the opposite is true for simple learning situations, where the scope of possible responses is restricted. Low anxiety may produce insufficient motivation, which may be inadequate to improve performance; and high anxiety may increase drive and motivation to a level that exceeds the optimal for a given task, and so interfere with the learning process and even lead to maladaptive responses. In other words, the differences between high-anxious and low-anxious children are particularly marked when the tasks are difficult or require creative solutions, or when the test situation is a threatening one. A classroom situation could become more threatening under various conditions, for example tests and examinations, the presence or absence of a person other than the tester (Cox, 1968), or the sex and the racial or cultural group of the tester, etc.

Guidelines, concerns and intentions

In the classroom and day-to-day life, one often comes across children with varying degree of adjustment problems, some of whom may be diagnosed as suffering from neurotic illness. Though a number of such children are highly anxious, one also finds individuals who do not show high anxiety. It is also a fact that there are numerous individuals who are reasonably well-adjusted and yet show high anxiety. One of the possible explanations could be that in the former case, the stresses and strains were perhaps too great and beyond the individual's capacity to cope, while in the latter case, the individual was not exposed to stresses and strains beyond the limits of their capability. In other words, it is apparent that apart from anxiety, circumstances and situations play an important part in bringing about the resultant behaviour, whether normal or abnormal. Anxiety which is associated with a state of apprehension, worry, sense of insecurity and the need for reassurance is largely anticipatory. Yet without some degree of anxiety in accord with reality, an individual would be without concern, even about events and things that are essential for survival and welfare. Morbid anxiety, however, overwhelms the individual and leads to a host of psychological problems.

Human relations with fellow human beings have a foundation in attitudes and beliefs which are part of the culture to which the person belongs. It therefore appears that when we interact, not only do we become conditioned to verbal and cognitive components of beliefs and attitudes, but also to verbal emotional reactions (Lokare, 1992). This kind of conditioning, like classical conditioning, through a process of generalisation, leads to semantic generalisation, creating the emotional components of beliefs and attitudes, as illustrated by Volkova (1953). Volkova's research suggests that we can pick up emotional components of prejudice through purely verbal means, without ever coming into contact with the object of our prejudice. For this reason, again it is vitally important that teachers, professional counsellors and therapists take account of this before reacting.

It should now be obvious that the process of human learning in this multicultural, multiracial world can create unforeseen complications and misunderstandings (and can turn living in this world into a nightmare for some). The risk of this happening is greater when, within a geographically-confined area, minorities within minorities live under the influence of the majority group which have their own, different cultures. Living together may help to bring about some form of integration, yet much of this could be superficial when one considers integration of immigrants and settlers within their own community, with its own religion, culture and beliefs. Remnants of old cultures continue to survive. Therefore, however willing, integration becomes a slow, complicated process, riddled with difficulties which could be further compounded by misdirected help that may cause additional (iatrogenic) problems (Lokare, 1992).

In investigating the needs of minority groups, one often fails to identify the real needs. The majority group, working with its own values and norms, uses these for comparison, instead of studying the minority group in its own right as a culture, and thus can, at times, fail to consider whether the minority group really has a particular need or wants help. It could be that the minority group wants help, but the type of help needed may be different from what the majority ethnic group thinks it to be (Lokare, 1992).

Although people have been vaguely aware of the importance of socio-cultural and socio-economic factors in problems of mental health, and of the need to provide everyone with a better emotional climate, lay people as well as professionals tend to have naive notions about this (Lokare, 1993). All this suggests that anxiety, which is a universal experience, is also a most important emotion from the teacher's and therapist's point of view, because of its effects on learning, achievement and adjustment. Anxiety is also a complex concept, and it involves an intricate and extremely complex relationship between other personality variables, biological inherited characteristics, cultural influences, the impact of education and the effects of different patterns of upbringing.

Hence, it should be borne in mind that if special arrangements are made for children from minority groups, then there is a risk of engendering feelings of inferiority, helplessness and insecurity in them, while fostering prejudices, stereotyping and so on in teachers, therapists and children of the majority group. In this way, things may go from bad to worse.

Our ability to identify the individual anxious child and the environmental stress that triggers anxiety, together with increased knowledge of its handling, is likely to be of greater practical value rather than concentrating solely on general characteristics, such as racial and cultural differences.

References

Angelino, H., Dollin, J. & Mech, E.V. (1956) 'Trends in the "fears and worries" of school children as revealed to socio-economic status and age', *Journal of Genetic Psychology*, 89, pp.263–76.

Brown, F.A. (1934) 'A psychoneurotic inventory for children nine and fourteen years of age', *Journal of Applied Psychology*, 19, pp.566–77.

Brown, F.A. (1936) 'A comparative study of the influence of race and locale upon emotional stability of children', *Journal of Genetic Psychology*, 49, pp.325–42.

Castaneda, A., McCandless, B.R. & Palermo, D.S. (1956) 'The children's form of the Manifest Anxiety Scale', *Child Development*, 27, pp.317–26.

Child, I.L. (1954) 'Personality', *Annual Review of Psychology*, 5, pp.149–70.

Colman, S.W., Mackay, D. & Fidell, B. (1972) 'English normative data on the Children's Manifest Anxiety Scale', *British Journal of Social and Clinical Psychology*, 2, pp.85–7.

Cox, F.N. (1960) 'Correlates of general and test anxiety in children', *Australian Journal of Psychology*, 12, pp.69–77.

Cox, F.N. (1968) 'Some relationships between test anxiety, presence or absence of male persons and boys' performance on a repetitive motor task', *Journal of Experimental Child Psychology*, 6, pp.11–12.

Dahlstrom, W.G. & Welsh, G.S. (1960) *An MMPI Handbook*, Minneapolis: Minnesota Press.

Drever, J. (1958) *A Dictionary of Psychology*, Harmondsworth: Penguin.

Durrett, M.A. (1965) 'Normative data on the Children's Manifest Anxiety Scale for Marathi-speaking Indian children on different income levels', *Indian Journal of Psychology*, 40, pp.1–6.

Essed, P. (1991) *Understanding Everyday Racism*, London: Sage Publications.

Eysenck, H.J. (1959) *Manual of the Maudsley Personality Inventory*, London: University of London Press.

Eysenck, H.J. (1967) *The Biological Basis of Personality*, Springfield, IL: Charles C. Thomas.

Eysenck, H.J. (1970) *The Structure of Human Personality*, London: Methuen.

Eysenck, S.B.G. (1965) *Manual of the Junior Eysenck Personality Inventory*, London: University of London Press.

Forsius, H. (1975) 'Special characteristics of children belonging to an ethnic minority', *Proceedings of the Fifth Conference of the Union of European Pedopsychiatrists*, Vienna: Verlag H. Egermann, pp.1,269–71.

Freud, S. (1955) 'The problems of anxiety', in Strachey, J. (ed.) *The Standard Edition of the Complete Psychological Works of Sigmund Freud*, Vol.XXII: 1932–1936, London: Hogarth Press, pp.81–111.

Gaudry, E.E. & Bradshaw, G.D. (1970) 'The differential effects of anxiety on performance in progressive and terminal school examinations', *Australian Journal of Psychology*, 22, pp.1–4.

Gorer, G. (1953) 'National character: Theory and practice', in Mead, M. & Me'traux, R. (eds) *Study of Culture at a Distance*, London: Pitman, pp.52–82.

Hebb, D.O. (1958) *A Text-Book of Psychology*, London: Saunders.

Heywood, H.C. & Dobbs, V. (1964) 'Motivation and anxiety in high school boys', *Journal of Personality*, 32, pp.371–9.

Hoch, P. & Zubin, J. (1950) *Anxiety*, New York: Grune and Stratton.

Horney, K. (1937) *The Neurotic Personality of Our Time*, New York: W.W. Norton.

Hull, C.L. (1943) *Principles of Behaviour*, New York: Appleton Century Crofts.

Jones, G.H. (1960) 'Learning and abnormal behaviour', in Eysenck, H.J. (ed.) *Handbook of Abnormal Psychology*, London: Pitman.

Joshi, M.C. & Singh, B. (1966) 'Influence of socio-economic background on the scores of some MMPI scales', *Journal of Social Psychology*, 70, pp.241–5.

Kapoor, S.D. (1964) 'Personality differences between the sexes', *Psychological Studies*, 9, pp.124–32.

Levitt, E.E. (1957) 'Ecological differences in performance on the CMAS', *Psychology Report*, 3, pp.281–6.

Lokare, V.G. (1966) 'The clinical application of a children's personality inventory', *Proceedings of the Sixth International Congress of Child Psychologists and Psychiatrists*, Edinburgh, unpublished.

Lokare, V.G. (1972a) 'The application of the Lokare's Modified Junior Maudsley Personality Inventory with particular reference to 8–12 year old children', *Journal of Child Psychology and Psychiatry*, 13, pp.37–46.

Lokare, V.G. (1972b) 'Neuroticism and extraversion on children as measured by the Lokare's Modified Junior Maudsley Personality Inventory', unpublished, MPhil. thesis.

Lokare, V.G. (1989) 'Anxiety in children: A cross-cultural perspective', in Varma, V.P. (ed.) *Anxiety in Children*, London and Sydney: Croom Helm.

Lokare, V.G. (1992) 'Respect for cultures, beliefs and attitudes: A way to better relationship and understanding', *Counselling Psychology Quarterly*, 5, pp.227–9.

Lokare, V.G. (1993) 'Counselling and the relevance of counsellors' and clients' views and attitudes', *British Journal of Guidance and Counselling*, 21, pp.41–5.

May, R. (1950) *The Meaning of Anxiety*, New York: Ronald Press.

McDougall, W. (1908) *An Introduction to Social Psychology*, London: Methuen.

McKeachie, W.J. & Doyle, C.L. (1966) *Psychology*, Reading, MA: Addison Wesley.

Mead, M. (1953) 'Study of culture at a distance', in Mead, M. & Me'traux, R. (eds) *Study of Culture at a Distance*, Chicago: University of Chicago Press.

Miller, N.E. & Dollard, J. (1941) *Social Learning and Imitation*, New Haven, CT: Yale University Press.

Montague, A. (1972) *Statement on Race*, New York: Oxford University Press.

Mowrer, O.H. (1939) 'A stimulus-response analysis of anxiety and its role as a reinforcing agent', *Psychological Review*, 46, pp.553–65.

Mowrer, O.H. (1950) *Learning Theory and Personality Dynamics*, New York: Ronald Press.

Nijhawan, H.K. (1972) *Anxiety in School Children*, New Delhi: Wiley Eastern Private.

Palermo, D.S. (1959) 'Racial comparison and additional normative data on the Children's Manifest Anxiety Scale', *Child Development*, 30, pp.53–7.

Pringle, M.L.K. & Cox, J. (1963) 'The influence of schooling and sex on test and general anxiety as measured by Sarason's Scales', *Journal of Child Psychology and Psychiatry*, 4, pp.157–65.

Rie, H.E. (1963) 'An exploratory study of the CMAS lie scale', *Child Development*, 34, pp.1,003–17.

Rosenberg, E. (1949) 'Anxiety and the capacity to bear it', *International Journal of Psycho-Analysis*, 30, pp.1–12.

Roycroft, C. (1968) *Anxiety and Neurosis*, London: Allen Lane.

Sarason, S.B. (1959) 'Test anxiety', *Journal of the National Educational Association*, 48, pp.26–7.

Sarason, S.B. & Mandler, G. (1952) 'Some correlates of test anxiety', *Journal of Abnormal and Social Psychology*, 47, pp.810–16.

Sarason, S.B., Davidson, K.S., Lighthall, F.F., Waite, R.R. & Ruebush, B.K. (1960) *Anxiety in Elementary School Children: A Report of Research*, New York: John Wiley.

Sinha, D. (1962) 'Cultural factors in emergence of anxiety', *Eastern Anthropologist*, 15, pp.21–37.

Springer, N.N. (1938) 'The influence of general social status on the emotional stability of children', *Journal of Genetic Psychology*, 53, pp.321–8.

Taylor, J.A. (1956) 'Drive theory and manifest anxiety', *Psychological Bulletin*, 53, pp.303–20.

Thompson, G.G. (1965) *Child Psychology*, Bombay: Times of India Press.

Volkova, U.D. (1953) 'On certain characteristics of conditioned reflexes to speech stimuli in children', *Fiziologiccheski Zurnal*, 39, pp.540–8.
Yerkes, R.M. & Dodson, J.D. (1908) 'The relationship of strength of stimulus to rapidity of habit-formation', *Journal of Comparative Neurology and Psychology*, 18, pp.459–82.

14 The management of school phobia

Sally Letts and Dino Cirelli

What is school phobia?

The problem starts with vague complaints of school and reluctance to attend, progressing to total refusal to go to school or remain in school in the face of persuasion, entreaty, recrimination and punishment. The behaviour may be accompanied by overt signs of anxiety or even panic. Characteristically, they remain at home with their parents' knowledge when they should be at school. (Hersov, 1977, cited in Blagg, 1990, p.121)

Hersov's diagnosis of school refusal (also referred to as 'school phobia') identifies clearly the nature and development of this very specific form of school non-attendance.

Despite the large number of papers and research programmes on school phobia in comparison to other childhood phobias, different opinions prevail among professionals as to its precise nature, causes and treatment (Miller et al., 1974). Reference to a group of children called 'neurotic' was made in Broadwin's 1932 study of truancy (cited in Baker & Wills, 1978), describing a special kind of truancy, distinguishing it from other forms of non-attendance. Partridge (1939, cited in Blagg, 1987) identified a group he labelled as 'psychoneurotic', who tended to be obedient, well-behaved, well-adjusted and generally liked school.

Johnson et al. (1941) first used the term 'school phobia', highlighting the role school played in contributing to extreme anxiety, the basis of which was the result of the child's fear of separating from its mother. Thereafter, 'school phobia' became a loose description of any school attendance problem based on an emotional disturbance with phobic tendencies. More recently, some writers, such as Hersov (1960), Khan and Nursten (1962) and Cooper (1966), felt the term 'school phobia' to be too specific, preferring instead the more inclusive term 'school refusal'. Blagg (1990) argued that this, unlike 'school phobia', fails to convey clearly to teachers and parents the emotions of fear, anxiety and helplessness which often accompany this condition. School refusal, he states, while being more inclusive, sounds less serious and could imply a *decision* not to attend school. Hsia (1984), in attempting to address the complexity of school non-attendance, conceptualised it as a continuum, from 'involuntary' symptoms at one end of the spectrum, where the child *cannot* go to school, to 'wilful' refusal at the other, where the child *will not* go. Various authors have attempted to dichotomise school phobia into groups: the neurotic or characterological (Coolidge et al., 1957, cited in Atkinson et al., 1985); Type 1 and Type 2, as differentiated by Kennedy (1965), and acute and chronic, as outlined by Berg et al. (1969). The former of each set occurs more suddenly and is generally easier to treat, while the latter is more gradual in onset and usually harder to deal with.

While these terms remain a source of confusion, differences between school phobia and truancy seem to be clearer, with school phobia being seen as one part of an anxiety disorder, and truancy as part of a conduct disorder (Hersov, 1960). Differentiation between these is vital, not only for purposes of identification, but more importantly, for treatment. It seems that while the motives for truancy may be many and complex, they rarely resemble the fear, anxiety and somatic distress of the phobic child (Goldenberg & Goldenberg, 1970, cited in McDonald & Shepherd, 1976). Truants tend to absent themselves without parental permission, and will not attend school because they do not want to. School phobics, however, usually remain at home with their parents' knowledge, and want to attend school but cannot, because they experience severe difficulty and emotional upset at this prospect.

Even this distinction, usually quite straightforward in pre-adolescence, may, according to Rubenstein and Hastings (1980), obscure the complexity of the problem in adolescence. Difficulties manifesting as school attendance problems may present as truancy, but could mask neurotic conflicts: often the genesis of school phobia. Perhaps the most useful working definition of the condition is that offered by Berg et al. (1969), identifying four important criteria:

1   severe difficulty in attending school, often leading to prolonged absences;
2   severe emotional upset, with excessive feelings of anxiety and fear, and complaints of feeling ill, without obvious organic cause;
3   staying at home with the knowledge of parents;
4   absence of significant antisocial disorders, such as stealing and lying.

Causes of school phobia

Various theoretical explanations have been proposed to account for the origins and causes of this condition. Perhaps the most influential is the psycho-analytic perspective, which sees the problem primarily as one of 'separation anxiety' (Eisenberg, 1958) – the result of a close, symbiotic mother–child relationship, in which the mother tends to be overprotective and the child excessively dependent. The psychodynamic perspective, while acknowledging the role of separation anxiety, seems to be too narrow an explanation, failing to account for the peak of school phobia between the ages of 11 and 13, and the fact that separating, in other environments, presented these children with few problems. Proposing the 'self-concept theory', Leventhal and Sills (1964) state that the child fears damaging an unrealistic self-image, which may have been excessively fostered at home, and subsequently feels threatened or attacked in the less personal setting of school, thus causing the child to avoid school and remain at home, where they are often held in high esteem. These expectations, while making the child vulnerable, may also strengthen their defensive behaviour and create a power issue with regard to school attendance.

While no specific behavioural theory of school phobia exists, since the early 1960s, learning theorists have suggested that school phobia may be the result of learnt maladaptive behaviour. They have seen the problem as either a simple fear of school or of separation (Garvey & Hegrenes, 1966), or a parenting management problem, in which the behaviour is maintained by secondary gains from the parents (Hersen, 1970). Their main focus has tended to concentrate on treatment, rather than cause, though considerable significance is placed on the part played by school-based factors, such as particular lessons, teachers and peers. Most recently, the Education Otherwise association has adopted a school-focused perspective, stressing the importance of school-based issues: they have interpreted school phobia as acute school-induced anxiety (Knox, 1989), and feel that the child should be removed from school and educated at home.

The diversity of theories would seem to reinforce the general view that school phobia is not one condition, but a group of conditions varying in severity and pathology (Blagg, 1990). Despite these varying emphases, all of the above would seem to identify and recognise certain common characteristics of school phobia: namely, an extreme reluctance to go to school, and/or extreme levels of anxiety towards some aspect of the school situation; this can be accompanied by somatic symptoms, which often dissipate once pressure to attend is removed.

The role of anxiety

In school phobia, the child often experiences feelings of extreme anxiety and/or fear of some aspect of the school situation, which they try to avoid. Anxiety, while seen as a normal reaction to stressful and dangerous situations, can become a problem when there is no real threat, or if it continues even after the causal event has passed. In school phobia, as in other phobias, anxiety may begin through a combination of factors: stress may arise from difficult situations, and/or life events, but it is the pupil's capacity to deal with such situations which is the deciding factor in whether or not the anxiety will become significant for them.

Anxiety, in its early stages, may manifest itself in a variety of ways: for example, stomach pains, sickness, headaches, coughs and sore throats. These somatic symptoms often have no organic cause. Clarification by medical professionals must be sought to ascertain whether these symptoms indicate real physical illness. In some instances, these symptoms may be the basis of a medical problem which can masquerade as an inability to attend school (Waller & Eisenberg, 1980; cited in Baker, 1990, p.155); the child may ultimately use this excuse for prolonged absence. In other children, it may result in withdrawn, fearful, apprehensive, irritable, aggressive or panicked behaviour at the prospect of going to school. This behaviour may be the result of realistic worries or irrational fears, or it may be precipitated by school-based situations such as a change of school, bullying, peer relationships, subjects or teachers, or home-based factors such as separation, family illness, deaths, sibling births, house moves or divorce. The inability of the parties to understand exactly what is happening in this situation will often create a reinforcing circle of confusion and anxiety between the child, parent and teachers as to the best way of dealing with it.

Treatment approaches

The basis of treatment of school phobia has tended to be guided by psycho-analytic/psychodynamic perspectives, focusing on insight and individual therapy, also stressing the importance of the mother–child relationship and fear of failure. The learning-theory perspective focuses on a variety of behavioural techniques, from both classical (flooding and desensitisation) and operant conditioning (contingency contracts and reinforcement) paradigms, stressing the importance of school-based factors. The family therapy perspective (Skynner, 1974; Hsia, 1984; Framrose, 1978; Bryce & Baird, 1986) has transcended the parent/child dyad, viewing school-phobic behaviour as systematic, protective and residing in the whole family. While acknowledging the role and importance of school-based factors in any treatment plan, this approach attempts to view family dysfunction by concentrating on the whole family unit and forces within the system which help to maintain the situation.

It has been suggested that the more successful treatments are those which transcend the psychodynamic/behavioural divide, using elements from each, in order to effectively address child, family and school factors (Blagg & Yule, 1984). An integrated approach to school phobia is one which recognises the importance of individual, family therapy, parent training, school, and home-based interventions. An effective model must be guided by some theoretical underpinning, and must also be flexible enough to address individual differences. Miller et al. (1974) suggest that whatever theoretical perspective one adheres to, treatment can be reduced to four essential elements:

1 a good relationship between the family, the child and the school;
2 clarification of real and/or imagined events causing the anxiety;
3 desensitising the fears through a variety of techniques to reduce anxiety;
4 early confrontation of the feared situation.

Assessment and interventions

The integrated approach outlined here draws upon various behavioural principles of conditioning and learning, but as Blagg clearly states:

> the search for a definitive behavioural technique or group of techniques to suit all cases is inappropriate. (Blagg & Yule, 1984, cited in Blagg, 1987, p.91)

The individualistic and heterogenous nature of the problem, both with respect to the causes of the difficulties and the way in which they are manifested, must be acknowledged. The issues giving rise to problems with a particular pupil are usually complex; this range and diversity of needs necessitates an individually-designed package which is unique to that pupil. Behavioural principles within a loose systems-based framework provide the most flexible and integrated response. Contingency management, social skills and cognitive approaches can be easily incorporated into the model.

For this model to function (see Figure 14.1), it is essential that certain key issues are addressed from the outset. An early response is always desirable, the overriding aim being to return the child to school as soon as is practically possible; thus it must be ascertained from the beginning whether the school placement is both appropriate to the pupil's needs

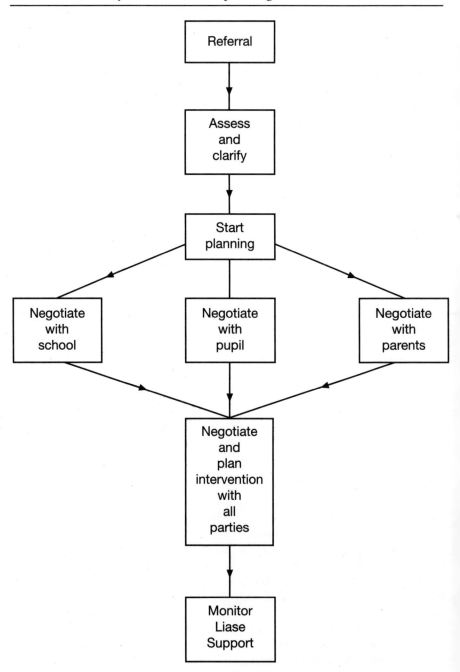

Figure 14.1   An integrated model of treatment for school phobia

and supported by their parents. Some indication of how long the difficulties have been evident will also be useful at this preliminary stage. Much
of this information can be obtained from the school and parents by the
school's education welfare officer, providing both a brief history and
background to the problem and a current picture. This information will
form the basis of the referral form, which will also indicate parental co-
operation and support for the referral, and detail any other professional
involvement – for example, the family GP and any other medical personnel who may have been contacted to investigate possible physical symptoms of illness.

The assessment is essentially an information-gathering exercise, and is
conducted through a series of face-to-face interviews and/or meetings
with all parties involved. The initial aim of this process is to collate
information and to establish contact and communication channels with all
key parties: the school, parents and child.

The assessment interviews usually begin with the 'link' teacher identified at the pupil's school. This will hopefully establish what facilities can
be made available for the pupil's return and how flexible the school
system is able to be in providing any resources required, for example
time, space, key personnel and limited timetables to cope with the
individual's needs. Preliminary contingency planning may also be discussed at this stage, in view of resource implications. To ensure that the
interviews remain as objective as possible, a pro forma is used, and
individual responses recorded. It is possible that several interviews may
be conducted with one or two link teachers. Information about the pupil
in and out of class situations and their relationships with other pupils is
recorded, building up a picture of the child's ability to function within the
school system, both currently and before the difficulties arose. Interviews
with school staff are also helpful in attempting to establish the school's
perspective on the problem and its abilities to respond to these kinds of
difficulties on a broad level and on an individual basis.

The parents are then invited, with their child, to an interview meeting
in the school. It is helpful if the parents are able to bring the pupil with
them at this stage. Arrangements should be made beforehand with the
school for the child to be accommodated after an initial meeting with the
interviewer. The parents are then interviewed, preferably together and
without their child. Again, the interviewer attempts to gain a broad
picture of the child, this time at home, looking at the background and
history of the difficulties and any possible 'trigger' factors in the child's or
family's history.

The interview attempts to clarify any issues for the parents and child,
real or perceived, past or present. The parents' perspective of the difficulties is crucial, and should be acknowledged. Hopefully, during this

process, the parents' willingness and ability to co-operate with the interviewer will be established. An opportunity for parents to tell their 'story' and to have the problem recognised is vital to building a good relationship. It is at this stage that the nature and purpose of the interviewer's involvement is explained, and that the aim and main objective of their role is a speedy return of the pupil to school, with the parents and school working actively with the child. Levels of motivation to aid the pupil's return should be apparent, and the interviewer should attempt to be as positive and encouraging as possible with all parties about the pupil's return to school.

By this stage, the interviewer or co-ordinator should have contacted any other professionals who may have been consulted about, or directly involved with, the pupil: the family GP, school nurse or social worker may be able to provide additional information which is relevant. If any questions or concerns remain about genuine illness, consultation must be sought and regular contact maintained. Inter-agency co-operation is as important as good working relationships between the major parties if any plan of management is to be agreed and effectively put into practice.

It is worthwhile considering the style and pace of interviews as well as their setting. Requests from any party should be taken seriously, and sensitivity to each party's perspective must be maintained. Once as much information as possible about the pupil has been gathered, the co-ordinator should arrange a meeting with the pupil in school. In this way, the co-ordinator is as prepared as possible and knows as much about the pupil's circumstances as is feasible at this stage. The meeting should take place in school, as this gives the pupil a clear message that a return is planned; it is less distracting than meeting in the family's home, more confidential, and may help the pupil to begin to engage. Within this remit, as much flexibility as possible should be offered. For example, the pupil may wish to meet after normal school hours, when other pupils have left, or away from the main teaching area. However, if it proves impossible for the child to attend their own school, an appropriate alternative meeting place may be offered. It is surprising how often a pupil is able to attend for this initial meeting, once its purpose has been made clear. If the pupil is only able to come into school with a parent, arrangements should be made beforehand to accommodate the parent for the duration of the interview.

This initial meeting should be brief – 15 minutes maximum – its sole purpose being to introduce the co-ordinator and to explain the aims of their involvement. Venues and agenda for subsequent meetings may be discussed, and some small task may be given to try to engage the pupil. It is essential, however, that content is kept low-key and non-threatening. It is important that the pupil understands that their views will be acknowledged, but it may take several meetings before the pupil's confidence can be gained sufficiently for them to speak of their worries and anxieties.

The co-ordinator should now have amassed much information and have begun to develop a relationship with the pupil. At this stage, they can begin to formulate some ideas about the management of this particular pupil's difficulties. Some prior negotiation with school and parents may now be necessary in addition to the ongoing meetings with the pupil: it will be useful to establish a 'baseline' for each party: issues they are willing and able to act upon and which are within their capability to change. This individual negotiation may be a rapid or lengthy process, depending on what is involved and the level and stage of the pupil's engagement.

All parties should then be brought together to formulate an action plan for the pupil's return. The plan must be negotiated by all, and confirm a clear role for each party, with specific tasks listed, and consensus on objectives. The action plan should then be written up and a copy given to each party. Contingency arrangements should also be made at this stage if the pupil is unable, for whatever reason, to reach one or all of the targets set. Clear means of liaison between the parties should also be written into this agreement. Regular review dates to monitor progress can also be set. Thus a managed programme of return has been established, and any breakdown can be reviewed and remedial action taken. The plan should be continually monitored and re-evaluated in the light of the pupil's progress.

Schools with little or no experience of a school-phobic pupil will usually welcome the opportunity to discuss issues of management at both an individual and whole-school level. Various strategies can be offered and have been found to be useful, but these will differ according to the individual resources and skills available within each particular school system. It must also be borne in mind that some school systems are, by their nature, more flexible than others. Useful strategies for the school may include:

- Appoint a linkperson for the pupil to turn to in addition to the co-ordinator. This may or may not be the same person designated as link teacher for the co-ordinator. What is important is that it is someone with whom the pupil feels comfortable and who is reasonably accessible to them.
- Set aside a 'refuge' or sanctuary of some kind, where the pupil is able to work outside the normal classroom environment, and where they may also spend unstructured times of the day when they feel most vulnerable. This could be a place such as the library or an activity such as helping a teacher prepare for lessons.

- Establish clear and effective communication within the school system, as well as with the co-ordinator. It is imperative that the link teacher is able to relay details about the pupil quickly to the rest of the staff group – the situation may change daily, and staff must be kept informed of developments so that they react appropriately.
- Use a limited or modified timetable, at least initially, allowing the pupil to suspend difficult or flashpoint areas – for example, a particular lesson, or assembly, or registration.
- The co-ordinator should be available easily and quickly to provide consultation to the school. A rapid response to a situation which may change is vital in supporting the school; frequent and close contact should facilitate this. The co-ordinator's help in investigating strategies with the school is seen as a practical and useful resource.

It is a key part of the co-ordinator's role to ensure that effective communication is established and continues. Without full co-operation and the continued support of all parties, it is impossible for the co-ordinator to work with the pupil. The assessment process will have indicated a number of issues which are a source of stress to the pupil and the family dynamics; these factors must be considered, if not addressed specifically. It is crucial that the parents feel involved, as all parties will be more motivated if they actively participate. Strategies which may be discussed with and useful to parents vary enormously, and will obviously be shaped by the findings of the assessment. These are some points which apply in most cases and have proven useful.

- Information about school phobia and anxiety in general may be useful for the parents, so that they understand what is happening to their child. Conveying the fact that school phobia usually occurs within 'good and caring' families often helps, as does the realisation that they are not alone, and that it can and does happen to other children. It is important that parents begin to feel in control of a situation which is usually outside their experience, rather than that they are handing their child over to a group of professionals to be 'treated' or 'fixed'. Working with parents will hopefully serve to empower rather than alienate them.

- It is important that the child is not encouraged in any way to remain at home. Parents are often unaware of the gains their child may receive while not attending school, for example more time on their own with mother, or opportunities to visit friends or relatives. Some clear guidelines as to what is expected of the parents while the child is being helped to re-establish attendance are useful. A written sheet of what the child's responsibilities are often helps to re-establish some element of control, and most parents find this encouraging and helpful.

● Help with establishing routines and practical arrangements should be offered. Often, parents have been dealing with their child's difficulties for some time in isolation, and as a result, may be extremely stressed, finding it has become difficult to maintain domestic routines. Some organisational help may be useful, and short-term modelling of 'good' parenting behaviour, particularly in setting and maintaining boundaries, is of great value. This will hopefully take pressure off parents in the short term, and also serve to reinforce their position.

Throughout the process of negotiation and planning with the school, parents and others, the relationship with the pupil is of paramount importance. The co-ordinator must engage the pupil in order to begin to clarify issues. It is important that the co-ordinator focuses initially on the pupil's strengths rather than the difficulties. Engagement of the pupil may be difficult and time-consuming, but is crucial to the process.

Essentially, a problem-solving approach is used to clarify the situations giving rise to anxiety. Steps can then be identified, and goals and objectives can be set up. It is important that throughout this process, the pupil is able to assume some control over the pace and means of return to school.

It is impossible to provide a comprehensive list of strategies to be employed with the pupil, but the following may prove useful.

● Offer some explanation of anxiety and why the pupil feels as they do. This is an attempt to 'normalise' the condition and allow the pupil to regain some control over their thoughts and feelings. Basic information about anxiety is important, and simple relaxation techniques can be taught and practised. Tapes are useful, and the pupil may practise relaxation either alone, with the co-ordinator or with a parent.

● Offer social skills training. This may include basic social skills or cover a specific area, such as assertiveness training or help with building self-esteem. This may help, for instance, in dealing with issues of bullying, or help in building up a friendship group.

● Offer specific counselling to deal with a particular issue, for example with bereavement. This may be undertaken by the co-ordinator or a specialist counsellor.

● Conduct desensitisation with the continued support of the co-ordinator, through a gradual and stepped return to school.

• Enlist the help of peers, either friends or other pupils with whom the pupil may have something in common. Something which is also useful but must be carefully handled is using the experience of another pupil who has successfully 'recovered' from school phobia.

Much material exists to help engage a pupil, and simple leaflets or tapes are always a useful back-up for the pupil to take away and follow up after a session with the co-ordinator.

Whatever issues are apparent for a school-phobic pupil, a co-ordinated approach with the support of all parties can bring about effective change. The initial assessment will provide a good starting point, and all information should be continually reviewed in the light of developments. Continual monitoring and evaluation of any programme ensures that issues are dealt with rapidly and effectively, ensuring a successful return to school.

Problem-solving

It may be useful to look at some common issues which arise among the three major parties, and to consider some ways of dealing with them.

Difficulties in engaging parents

School phobia can often cause confusion and distress among parents. In some instances, these feelings can temporarily disable them from engaging actively. Hesitancy and inactivity may be interpreted as lack of motivation, though very often, they may be the result of the family's fear of being judged, thought of as bad, inadequate or of losing control. Bandler and Grinder (1975, cited in Kingston, 1984) suggest that motivation is often wrongly changed from a process into an entity, implying that families are either motivated or not; in fact, everyone is motivated (to fulfil wishes and interests and to reduce conflicts), though this may be affected by the context in which it occurs:

• Explore the reason for the referral and its route. Was it voluntary or enforced?
• Ensure that the first meeting takes place away from the home, preferably in school.
• Build up an understanding of the parents' view of the situation. Ascertain the parents' level of consensus and their view of the importance of school attendance.
• Explain your role, aims and the purpose of involvement.

Lack of co-operation

This model of management is based upon collaboration, emphasising the importance of parental roles and responsibilities. Will (1983) points out that lack of collaboration may occur either when the family is too anxious (where the fear of change outweighs the cost of not changing), or when there is too little anxiety, causing them to become resistant and rigid:

- Acknowledge the family's concerns and ambivalence; tentatively empathise with their feelings (anxiety, fear, apprehension, etc.).
- Explain and clarify your aims and objectives; provide information about how you intend to work, and the process of involvement.
- Reframe the school phobia by 'normalising' the condition through stories and reflections on work with similar situations.
- Explore the advantages of continued school attendance, with particular emphasis upon the educational and social implications.
- Encourage ideas and suggestions of what the family believe might help change the situation.
- Give realistic hope that the difficulty can be overcome; to this end, success or failure may ultimately rest heavily upon the persistent determination and conviction on the part of the co-ordinator (Framrose, 1978).
- Consider and explore the options available, including the possible legal implications; Skynner (1974) proposes that in adopting a role of 'real authority', the co-ordinator is merely attempting to clarify and make explicit what are, in effect, the real possibilities and consequences of continued non-attendance.

Responding to setbacks

Despite detailed planning, setbacks are a feature of school phobia. The effect of setbacks will be dependent upon their timing and the fact that parties may be unprepared for them:

- Develop contingency arrangements for successive stages of the planned return to school.
- Respond to each situation quickly; be available for the family, pupil and school.
- Discuss and identify possible causes of the setback.
- Deal with practical problems, if possible.
- Acknowledge and consolidate progress to date; motivate and encourage the parties to proceed.
- Renegotiate subsequent targets; if necessary, make the targets smaller, more manageable, and above all, achievable.

- Provide encouragement and praise for success, however small.
- Consider referral to specialist agencies (e.g. the Child and Family Consultation Service) to address extreme and serious breakdowns in family functioning.

Parents unable to establish and maintain routines

Successful management of school phobia depends on establishing and implementing consistent and practical routines on school days:

- Explore and clarify with the parents details of daily routines.
- Identify problem areas with these routines.
- Confirm individual roles and responsibilities.
- Identify the suitability and availability of additional support (education welfare officers, teachers, relatives, neighbours, friends) to assist with routines.
- Establish clear guidelines for the parents if the child is unable to attend school and/or remains at home.
- Agree that the parents are to inform the school and the co-ordinator as soon as possible if the child is absent for any reason.
- If the child remains at home but is well enough to attend school, the parents should limit access to television, games, toys, etc., which may provide secondary gains for remaining at home.

Parents in conflict with professionals

Parents may already have come into contact with numerous professionals or agencies; this may give rise to conflicting information and views being expressed, leading the family to challenge professionals:

- Renegotiate aims and objectives with the parties.
- Ensure regular communication and liaison between the parties.
- Provide a clear plan of action.

Engaging the reluctant or silent pupil

Successful and productive work with children is dependent upon establishing a secure and trusting relationship. This is no simple task, and will take time. A relationship is assisted by an empathic and sensitive approach which is non-threatening, real, and takes account of the child's age and development. It is important to acknowledge issues of power and control. The child may be reluctant, and unable to see any purpose in engaging.

The silent pupil can be difficult to work with. Increased frustration can lead to asking more and more questions. In an attempt to 'get through', it is possible to talk too much, and subsequently fail to listen:

- Write to the child, inviting them to attend a meeting.
- Pay attention to practical arrangements, such as ensuring rooms in school are comfortable and free from interruption. Make the child feel as relaxed as possible.
- Briefly explain your role and the purpose of your involvement.
- Keep the focus on getting to know the child and not the problem. Work at the child's pace.
- Keep initial meetings brief.
- Use concrete tools to aid communication, such as worksheets, games, drawings, etc.
- Ensure agreed meetings are kept and begin on time, in order to provide security and predictability for the child.
- If the child is unable to meet in school, consider changing the venue for meetings to a more neutral base. Use the home as the last resort.
- After the meeting, write to the child thanking them for attending and suggesting a new date to meet again.
- Remain calm: try not to ask too many questions. The child may sense your frustration through your tone of voice and expression.
- Think out loud: explain what you are doing and why; explain what they are doing and why. Be tentative in your interpretations: they may be wrong.
- Consider social tasks, for example a walk around the school.
- Interpret the silence; attend to non-verbal expressions or gestures, simply repeating what is observed. This may prompt the child to agree or correct your observation.
- If appropriate, share experiences of your work with other pupils having difficulties.

The child has difficulties with peer relationships/bullying

The nature of school phobia may significantly undermine a child's confidence and self-image. Very often, it is their inability to cope with the social context of the school environment which causes anxiety and possible withdrawal from situations. These feelings may have been caused and exacerbated by experiences both in and out of school when the child may have been bullied (physically or verbally).

Dealing with these difficulties can be problematic, and will be easier within a relationship where the child feels safe, secure and understood:

- Take allegations seriously, and investigate them.
- Identify areas of concern and details of incidents.
- If appropriate and helpful, attend to practical arrangements (e.g. change of groups, tutor/subject groups, sanctuary arrangements for break/lunch/home times).
- Ensure that the child's physical safety is secured.
- Undertake individual work on identifying strategies to help deal with these situations. Rehearse them and put them into action.
- Identify levels of concern in specific situations.

The child may become dependent upon the co-ordinator

Effective management of school phobia requires intensive, sometimes daily contact with the child and the family. Over a period of time, the relationship, if successful, becomes very significant for the child:

- Constantly monitor your role. Be aware of the child's needs and the importance of boundaries and professionalism.
- Ensure that regular consultation is available to explore your aims and objectives.
- Agree a clear contract between the co-ordinator, child and family. Ensure that this contract is reviewed regularly.
- Negotiate 'endings', and work towards these, unless the situation breaks down unexpectedly.

Limited resources

Successful re-integration is dependent on the flexibility of resources and the co-operation of the school. Close links with a member of staff, possible exemption in the short term from certain areas of the curriculum, the use of withdrawal facilities, part-time attendance and a change of tutor or subject groups may be helpful. The ability to meet these needs will vary from one school to another. In order to establish an individual plan of action, availability and provision of these facilities needs to be clarified at the assessment stage. Recommendations may need to be communicated, both to staff in general and to other relevant educational support services (e.g. education welfare officers):

- Offer ongoing support and consultation to the school.
- Ensure the involvement of senior personnel who can arrange provisions.
- Explore with the link teacher any support services available to the school that may not yet have been utilised.

- Ensure that details of any planned return are communicated to all relevant members of staff.

Conclusion

The integrated approach outlined here is not intended to be a comprehensive account of school phobia; however, it does attempt to recognise the different causes and complexity of this condition. This model indicates that thorough assessments, clear planning and individual treatment packages provide useful frameworks for planning strategies for the successful management of school phobia.

References

Atkinson, L., Quarrington, J. & Cyr, J.J. (1985) 'School refusal: The heterogeneity of a concept', *American Journal of Orthopsychiatry*, 55(1), pp.83–101.

Baker, H. (1990) 'The management of school phobia', in Gupta, R.M. & Coxhead, P. (eds) *Intervention with Children*, London and New York: Routledge.

Baker, H. & Wills, U. (1978) 'School phobia: Classification and treatment', *British Journal of Psychiatry*, 132, pp.492–9.

Bandler, R. & Grinder, J. (1975) *The Structure of Magic*, Vol.1, Palo Alto, CA: Science and Behaviour Books.

Berg, I., Nichols, K. & Pritchard, C. (1969) 'School phobia: Its classification and relationship to dependency', *Journal of Child Psychology and Psychiatry*, 10, pp.123–41.

Blagg, N.R. (1987) *School Phobia and its Treatment*, London: Croom Helm.

Blagg, N. (1990) 'School phobia', in Lane, D.A & Miller, A. (eds) *School Phobia in Child and Adolescent Therapy: A Handbook*, Buckingham: Open University Press, pp.120–37.

Blagg, N. & Yule, W. (1984) 'The behavioural treatment of school refusal: A comparative study', *Behaviour Research and Therapy*, 22, pp.119–27.

Broadwin, I.T. (1932) 'A contribution to the study of truancy', *American Journal of Orthopsychiatry*, 2, pp.253–9.

Bryce, G. & Baird, D. (1986) 'Precipitating a crisis: Family therapy and adolescent school refusers', *Journal of Adolescence*, 9, pp.199–213.

Coolidge, J., Hahn, P. & Peck, A. (1957) 'School phobia: Neurotic crisis or way of life', *American Journal of Orthopsychiatry*, 27, pp.296–306.

Cooper, M.G. (1966) 'School refusal', *Educational Research*, 8(2), pp.115–27.

Eisenberg, L. (1958) 'School phobia: A study in the communication of anxiety', *American Journal of Psychiatry*, 114, pp.712–18.

Framrose, R. (1978) 'Outpatient treatment of severe school phobia', *Journal of Adolescence*, 1, pp.353–61.

Garvey, W.P. & Hegrenes, J.R. (1966) 'Desensitisation techniques in the treatment of school phobia', *American Journal of Orthopsychiatry*, 36, pp.147–52.

Goldenberg, H. & Goldenberg, I. (1970) 'School phobia: Childhood neurosis or learned maladaptive behaviour?', *Exceptional Children*, 37, pp.220–6.

Hersen, M. (1970) 'Behaviour modification approach to a school phobia case', *Journal of Clinical Psychology*, 26, pp.128–32.

Hersov, L. (1960) 'Refusal to go to school', *Journal of Child Psychology and Psychiatry*, 1, pp.137–45.

Hersov, L. (1977) 'School refusal', in Rutter, M. & Hersov, L. (eds) *Child and Adolescent Psychiatry: Modern Approaches*, Oxford: Blackwell.

Hsia, H. (1984) 'Structural and strategic approach to school phobia/school refusal', *Psychology in the Schools*, 21, pp.360–7.

Johnson, A.M., Falstein, E.K., Szurek, S. & Svendsen, M. (1941) 'School phobia', *American Journal of Orthopsychiatry*, 11, pp.702–11.

Kennedy, W.A. (1965) 'School phobia: Rapid treatment of fifty cases', *Journal of Abnormal Psychology*, 70(4), pp.285–9.

Khan, J. & Nursten, J. (1962) 'School refusal: A comprehensive view of school phobia and other failures of school attendance', *American Journal of Orthopsychiatry*, 32, pp.707–18.

Kingston, P. (1984) 'But they aren't motivated', *Journal of Family Therapy*, 6, pp.381–403.

Knox, P. (1989) 'Home based education: An alternative approach to "school phobia" ', *Educational Review*, 41(2), pp.143–50.

Leventhal, T. & Sills, M. (1964) 'Self image in school phobia', *American Journal of Orthopsychiatry*, 34(4), pp.685–95.

McDonald, J.E. & Shepherd, G. (1976) 'School phobia: An overview', *Journal of School Psychology*, 14(4), pp.291–306.

Miller, L.C., Barrett, C.L. & Hampe, E. (1974) 'Phobias of childhood in a pre-scientific era', in Davies, A. (ed.) *Child Personality and Psychopathology: Current Topics* (Vol.1), New York: John Wiley, pp.89–134.

Partridge, J.M. (1939) 'Truancy', *Journal of Mental Science*, 85, pp.45–81.

Rubenstein, J.S. & Hastings, E.M. (1980) 'School refusal in adolescence: Understanding the symptom', *Adolescence*, 15(60), pp.775–81.

Skynner, A.C. (1974) 'School phobia: A reappraisal', *British Journal of Medical Psychology*, 47, pp.1–17.

Waller, D. & Eisenberg, L. (1980) 'School refusal in childhood: A psychiatric, paediatric perspective', in Hersov, L. & Berg, I. (eds) *Out of School*, New York: John Wiley.

Will, D. (1983) 'Some techniques for working with resistant families of adolescents', *Journal of Adolescence*, 6, pp.13–26.

Will, D. & Baird, D. (1984) 'An integrated approach to dysfunction in inter-professional systems', *Journal of Family Therapy*, 6, pp.275–90.

15 Anxiety associated with learning disabilities

Chinta Mani

In general, there has been insufficient research into specific psychiatric disorders in the context of learning disabilities to draw firm conclusions about their incidence and prevalence. Interpretation of the studies available so far must be cautious, because of the lack of uniform criteria, and possible interviewer bias.

Several studies have reported a higher incidence of anxiety disorders in people with learning disabilities than in those without them (Malpass et al., 1960; Feldhusen & Klausmeier, 1962; Cochrane & Cleland, 1963). Tredgold and Soddy (1956) examined psychoneuroses among people with learning disabilities, and regarded hysterical manifestations as the most frequent, followed by anxiety states and obsessive-compulsive reactions. Ollendick and Ollendick (1982) reported that anxiety states and phobic disorders were quite common in people with learning disabilities, both in hospital and outpatient settings. The higher incidence of anxiety in mentally handicapped people can be explained because of their social and educational failure, institutionalisation, lack of communication and articulation, and their emotional immaturity.

Webster (1963) studied 159 children with learning disabilities between the ages of 3 and 6, and concluded that all of them had some emotional disturbance. Richardson et al. (1979) followed up 222 children with learning disabilities from birth to 22 years of age, and concluded that 26% suffered from neurotic problems and another 20% from conduct and antisocial problems. The frequency was highest for those with IQs of less than 50. Craft (1959) studied 324 mentally handicapped inpatients, and reported that 33% could be diagnosed as having 'personality disorders', with anxiety as a prominent feature.

Some people believe that limited awareness of difficulties protects a mentally handicapped person from distress and anxiety. Despite this, a significant number of children with learning disabilities suffer from

235

neurotic problems. Rutter et al. (1970) reported an increase in neurotic and conduct disorders in children with learning disabilities. Corbett (1979) concluded that 4% of severely mentally handicapped children in his Camberwell survey suffered from neurotic disorders. It is possible to diagnose neurotic disorders in mentally handicapped children, even in those with a severe degree of mental handicap, although it is not possible to do so in profoundly mentally handicapped children (Reid, 1982).

Manifestations

Disorders in which anxiety forms the predominant feature are:

- panic disorder;
- generalised anxiety disorder;
- obsessive-compulsive disorder;
- phobic disorders (e.g. agoraphobia, social phobia and simple phobia);
- post-traumatic stress disorder.

The clinical presentation in people with learning disabilities is anything but typical, and the frequent manifestations of anxiety are as follows:

- *Symptoms*
  - excessive worrying;
  - marked self-conciousness;
  - separation anxiety;
  - abdominal pain;
  - somatic complaints;
  - headaches;
  - sleep disturbance;
  - hyperventilation, etc.

- *Signs*
  - worried look;
  - tics;
  - signs of autonomic overactivity (e.g. tremors, palpitations and sweating, inattention, distractibility, reluctance to speak and mannerisms, etc.).

- *Behaviour*
  - fearfulness;
  - social withdrawal;
  - tension;

- restlessness;
- irritability;
- self-injurious behaviour;
- regression in toilet habits (e.g. enuresis and encopresis);
- acting out and attention-seeking behaviour (e.g. aggression, temper tantrums or absconding, etc.).

Separation anxiety may manifest as somatic syptoms, and may lead to school refusal. Phobic anxiety may manifest as specific fears, such as dog phobia. Underlying anxiety may be the cause of various conduct and behavioural problems, and may be related to difficulties at home and at school.

The interviewer may face special difficulties while talking to patients with learning disabilities, because of their poor communication, and may have to ask questions in a very simple and concrete way. Frequently, not much history is available from the patient, and therefore more reliance has to be given to the account given by carers. Physical signs of anxiety are more useful in such circumstances. Some therapists use the method of direct observation of the child's behaviour in the presence of real or simulated anxiety-producing stimuli; however, this latter approach may be considered unethical by others. The possibility of observers' bias and the likelihood of the child changing their behaviour while under observation must be borne in mind. Observation of the child in a natural situation is preferable but more time-consuming. Observations in a simulated setting may become necessary when anxiety does not occur very frequently.

Aetiological factors

There are several factors which contribute to causation of anxiety in children with learning disabilities, and there are several theories to explain the genesis of anxiety.

Cerebral damage

Brain damage may result in below-average intelligence, which impairs socially-adaptive behaviour in terms of maturation, learning and social adjustment (Robinson & Robinson, 1965).

The development of self-care skills, such as feeding, walking, talking, habit training and interaction with peers, is delayed in children with learning disabilities, and this clashes with parental expectations, leading to heightened anxiety in both the parents and children, and a sense of failure in the children.

The presence of limitations in the learning process, particularly if associated with sensory handicaps such as deafness or blindness, deprives mentally handicapped children of appropriate learning experiences. In many, the mental handicap is also associated with poor motivation, distractibility, poor memory and poor general ability, and all these contribute to the sense of failure and anxiety in learning situations.

Learning theories

The principles of learning theories apply equally to people with learning disabilities, and these assume that anxiety is a learnt behaviour in the following ways:

- The stimulus-response model, based on the work of Pavlov (1941) and Wolpe (1958), assumes that anxiety is a classically-conditioned response to environmental or cognitive stimuli.
- The social learning model, based on the work of Bandura (1968), assumes that anxiety is precipitated and maintained by cognitive factors associated with external stimuli, and that it is an active or dynamic process, rather than a form of passive association.
- The response-reinforcement model assumes that anxiety is maintained by the consequences of an anxiety reaction.

There are some limitations to these models, particularly when applied to children with learning disabilities. Some basic responses are essential for learning, and as learning proceeds, these responses are modified. Many mentally handicapped children have a limited repertoire of responses. Also, because of their inattention, hyperactivity and behavioural problems, they are unable to interpret cues in their environment correctly, and this hinders their learning and maintains the anxiety.

Social learning theory

This theory hypothesises that because they have more experience of failure, children with learning disabilities have less expectancy for success, which increases their anxiety. Stevenson and Zigler (1958) found that mentally handicapped children were more anxious and performed poorly, and they postulated that anxiety was a consequence of poor performance, rather than the cause of it.

Psychodynamic theory

Development of personality has not been widely studied in children with learning disabilities. Nevertheless, the principles of psychodynamic theories apply equally. Freud postulated that the personality consists of the id, which includes basic instincts; the ego, which develops from the id and is concerned with testing reality and bringing basic instincts into line with reality; and the superego, which develops through interaction with environments and is concerned with determining social values and behaviour. Anxiety results from a conflict between the id and the ego on the one hand, and the ego and the superego on the other.

It is thought that formulation of the ego is defective in people with learning disabilities, and that this leads to impaired function of the superego. This further leads to poor development of the psychological defence mechanisms required to deal with anxiety and guilt.

Cobb (1961) hypothesised that children with learning disabilities have difficulties in primitive differentiation, integration and generalisation, and that this impairs the ability of the ego to deal with the environment effectively. Robinson and Robinson (1965) stated that people with mental handicap are seriously handicapped in their ability to handle the demands of the id and the superego in the context of the real world because of their defective ego. Lack of normal development of the ego interferes with the ability to grasp reality and comprehend and anticipate the consequences of one's actions.

Delay in reaching developmental milestones is associated with delay in resolving psychodynamic conflicts at every stage of psychological development, such as giving up bottle feeding, gaining control of the bowels and bladder, and working out the Oedipal complex. Anxiety and insecurity results, depending upon the level of mental handicap and the ability of parents or carers to handle it. A mentally handicapped child who finds it difficult to control aggressive impulses will experience more anxiety.

Treatment

General principles of treatment are the same as for children with normal intelligence, although there have been few specific studies in the field of learning disabilities. Stress must be laid on multidisciplinary input from teachers, nurses, psychologists, social workers and families. The person's limitations should be accepted, and treatment goals should be realistic, given the degree of learning disabilities.

Drug treatment

Three types of drugs have been used for the treatment of anxiety: beta-adrenergic blockers, benzodiazepines and, over recent years, Buspiriline.

These can be combined with other psychological treatments, and help to make people more amenable to them.

Benzodiazepines are most commonly used, and are more effective in reducing anxiety than placebo (Soloman & Hart, 1978). Valium and Librium have been widely used, including in people with mild learning disabilities. However, their side effects, such as paradoxical aggression, unsteadiness on the feet, drowsiness and slowing of psychomotor skills, can be more troublesome in persons with learning disabilities.

Beta-adrenergic drugs such as Propranalol are helpful when anxiety is manifested in physical features such as sweating, tremors, palpitations, diarrhoea and frequency of micturition. These are also effective in panic and generalised anxiety states.

Buspiriline is only a recent addition to the range of anti-anxiety drugs, and is claimed to be free of side effects of sedation and addiction. However, its role in the field of learning disabilities, and particularly in children, has not been well researched. Nevertheless, it remains an important option, either with or without other drugs.

In highly-anxious patients, and in circumstances where anxiety is associated with severe aggression, temper tantrums and disruptive behaviour, the use of major tranquillisers such as Thioridazine in very small doses is justified. If anxiety is associated with depression, then use of antidepressant medication alone or in combination with anxiolytics should be considered.

Anxiety usually responds to drug treatment alone, or in combination with other psychological measures. It is very important to address the interpersonal and family problems contributing to anxiety. Drugs should not be used indiscriminately. However, they should not be avoided if their use is considered justifiable on clinical grounds. Finally, some limitations in goals have to be accepted, as it may not be possible to change an established pattern of a person's behaviour and interaction with their family and other carers.

Behaviour treatments

These are based on the principles of learning theories which assume that after the onset of anxiety through classical or operant conditioning, it is maintained by repeated reassurance and the attention given to the child from the carers. There are two main techniques available.

Systematic desensitisation

In this method, the child is first trained in deep muscle relaxation, which is an antagonistic response to anxiety. Once in a relaxed state, the child is presented with anxiety-provoking stimuli, starting with least anxiety-provoking, and gradually proceeding in stages to most anxiety-provoking. The stimuli are presented either in the imagination or in real-life situations. This method is very effective in the treatment of anxiety and fear in adults and children with normal intelligence. However, its use in persons with learning disabilities has not been well documented through research. Ability to gain full relaxation and imagine anxiety-provoking stimuli is very limited in people with learning disabilities, due to impaired cognition. However, this technique could be helpful in people with mild or moderate learning disabilities.

Modelling

This is based on the theory of vicarious learning, and is of three types: filmed modelling, live modelling and participant modelling.

In filmed modelling, the patient watches a series of films in which a model performs progressively more intimate interaction with the stimuli which would give anxiety to the patient. In live modelling, the patient observes the model interacting with real-life anxiety-provoking situations, while in participant modelling, the patient observes the model, and also participates in the interaction with support from the therapist, thus trying to overcome their anxiety.

These behavioural techniques are considered very useful in treating anxiety and fear. However, their use in people with learning disabilities has limitations, and more research is needed, particularly with children. Combined with judicious use of medication, these are potentially strong treatment tools.

Social skills training

Generally speaking, people with learning disabilities lack the interpersonal and social skills necessary to relate to peers and everyday life situations. This often leads to their rejection by peers, and this perpetuates anxiety and avoidance behaviour, which consequently maintains anxiety.

Therefore, it is very important to pay due attention to the teaching of skills like assertiveness, ability to initiate and hold good conversations, sharing, co-operation and other socially desirable behaviours when dealing with others. These skills are necessary in reducing anxiety in interpersonal situations and increasing the confidence and quality of life of people with learning disabilities. However, teaching these skills to those with moderate or severe learning disabilities can be very difficult and frustrating, and a lot of perseverance and patience is required on the part of carers and teachers.

Conclusion

The prevalence of anxiety is high in children with learning disabilities, because of the associated cognitive and other deficits. The manifestations of anxiety are varied, and diagnosis based on interview alone is difficult and not always possible. The questions should be simple, so that the patient can understand them, and more emphasis has to be given to reports from the carers.

The general principles of management are the same as in children without learning disabilities, but more tolerance and perseverance is required on the part of the therapist and the carers, and therapeutic goals have to be realistic, depending upon the degree of learning disabilities. Finally, more research is needed in this field.

References

Bandura, A. (1968) 'Modeling approaches to the modification of phobic disorders', in Porter, R. (ed.) *Ciba Foundation Symposium: The Role of Learning in Psychotherapy*, London: Churchill, pp.201–23.

Cobb, H.V. (1961) 'Self-concept of the mentally retarded', *Rehabilitation Records*, 2, pp.21–5.

Cochrane, I.L. & Cleland, C.C. (1963) 'Manifest anxiety of retardates and normals matched as to academic achievement', *American Journal of Mental Deficiency*, 67, pp.539–42.

Corbett, J.A. (1979) 'Psychiatric morbidity and mental retardation', in James, F.E. & Smith, R.P. (eds) *Psychiatric Illness and Mental Handicap*, London: Gaskell Press, pp.11–26.

Craft, M. (1959) 'Mental disorder in the defective: A psychiatric survey among inpatients', *American Journal of Mental Deficiency*, 63, pp.829–34.

Feldhusen, J.F. & Klausmeier, H.J. (1962) 'Anxiety, intelligence and achievement in children of low, average and high intelligence', *Child Development*, 33, pp.403–9.

Malpass, L.F., Mark, S. & Palermo, D.S. (1960) 'Responses of retarded children to the Children's Manifest Anxiety Scale', *Journal of Educational Psychology*, 51(5), pp.305–8.

Ollendick, T.H. & Ollendick, D.G. (1982) 'Anxiety disorders', in Matson, J.L. & Barrett, R.P. (eds) *Psychopathology in the Mentally Retarded*, London and New York: Grune and Stratton, pp.77–119.

Pavlov, I.P. (1941) *Conditioned Reflexes and Psychiatry*, New York: International Publishers.

Reid, A.H. (1982) *The Psychiatry of Mental Handicap*, London: Blackwell Scientific Publications.

Richardson, S.A., Katz, M., Keller, H., McLaren, L. & Rubinstein, B. (1979) 'Some characteristics of a population of mentally retarded young adults in a British city: A basis for estimating some service needs', *Journal of Mental Deficiency Research*, 23(4), pp.275–83.

Robinson, H.B. & Robinson, N.M. (1965) *The Mentally Retarded Child: A Psychological Approach*, New York: McGraw-Hill.

Rutter, M., Tizard, J. & Whitmore, K. (1970) *Education, Health and Behaviour*, London: Longman.

Soloman, K. & Hart, R. (1978) 'Pitfalls and prospects in clinical research on antianxiety drugs: Benzodiazepines and placebo – A research review', *Journal of Clinical Psychiatry*, 61, pp.823–9.

Stevenson, H.W. & Zigler, E.F. (1958) 'Probability learning in children', *Journal of Experimental Psychology*, 56(3), pp.185–92.

Tredgold, R.F. and Soddy, K. (1956) *A Textbook of Mental Deficiency* (9th edn), London: Bailliere, Tindall and Cox.

Webster, T. (1963) 'Problems of emotional development in young retarded children', *American Journal of Psychiatry*, 120, July, pp.37–43.

Wolpe, J. (1958) *Psychotherapy by Reciprocal Inhibition*, Stanford, CA: Stanford University Press.

Index

Coping
with
Children
in
Stress

edited by Ved Varma

Childhood is a time of rapid change which can cause stress for many children, but those with special needs may have to face additional stresses, either at home or at school. This book investigates how to handle children with stresses derived from various sources – health, educational and social – looking at the causes and effects of stress, ways of preventing or minimising it, as well as coping strategies. The chapters focus on children with sensory impairments, physical disabilities, learning difficulties, emotional or behavioural difficulties, as well as gifted children and those from ethnic minorities.

This book is essential reading not only for special needs teachers but also for mainstream teachers of all age-ranges.

Ved Varma was formerly an educational psychologist with the Institute of Education, University of London, the Tavistock Clinic, and for the London Boroughs of Richmond and Brent.

1996   179 pages   Hbk   1 85742 252 X   £16.95
Pbk   1 85742 253 8   £32.50
Price subject to change without notification

arena

Promoting Positive Parenting

A professional guide to establishing groupwork
programmes for parents of children with behavioural
problems

David Neville, Dick Beak and Liz King

In association with the Centre for Fun & Families

In the long term, physical punishment does not work with children. It demeans both the child and the parents. A range of other methods are needed ... It is my hope that this book will be an invaluable guide to professional staff who work with parents to try a new and very positive approach to help them with the hardest but most rewarding job in the world – being a 'positive parent'. Sue Townsend

The Centre for Fun and Families is a national voluntary organisation which was established in 1990. Its objective is to empower parents who are experiencing behaviour and communication difficulties with their children. This book both shares with the reader the theoretical ideas that underpin the work of the Centre and provides a practical guide of how to undertake such a programme, thereby enabling the reader to react sensitively and productively to the unforeseen circumstances which are inevitable when running a groupwork programme. Professionals coming to these methods for the first time can work through the text safe in the knowledge that these are tried and tested ways of working, which are known to be effective. At a time when attention is focused on the importance of parenting and the way in which children are brought up, no practitioner working with this field should ignore the message within these covers.

1995   160 pages   1 85742 266 X   £14.95

Price subject to change without notification

arena